WOMEN'S ISSUES

NEW RESEARCH ON BREASTFEEDING AND BREAST MILK

WOMEN'S ISSUES

Additional books and e-books in this series can be found on Nova's website under the Series tab.

WOMEN'S ISSUES

NEW RESEARCH ON BREASTFEEDING AND BREAST MILK

KAI SANTOS MELO
EDITOR

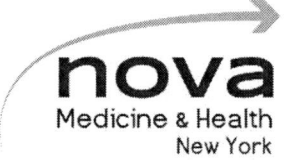

Copyright © 2020 by Nova Science Publishers, Inc.

All rights reserved. No part of this book may be reproduced, stored in a retrieval system or transmitted in any form or by any means: electronic, electrostatic, magnetic, tape, mechanical photocopying, recording or otherwise without the written permission of the Publisher.

We have partnered with Copyright Clearance Center to make it easy for you to obtain permissions to reuse content from this publication. Simply navigate to this publication's page on Nova's website and locate the "Get Permission" button below the title description. This button is linked directly to the title's permission page on copyright.com. Alternatively, you can visit copyright.com and search by title, ISBN, or ISSN.

For further questions about using the service on copyright.com, please contact:
Copyright Clearance Center
Phone: +1-(978) 750-8400   Fax: +1-(978) 750-4470   E-mail: info@copyright.com

NOTICE TO THE READER

The Publisher has taken reasonable care in the preparation of this book, but makes no expressed or implied warranty of any kind and assumes no responsibility for any errors or omissions. No liability is assumed for incidental or consequential damages in connection with or arising out of information contained in this book. The Publisher shall not be liable for any special, consequential, or exemplary damages resulting, in whole or in part, from the readers' use of, or reliance upon, this material. Any parts of this book based on government reports are so indicated and copyright is claimed for those parts to the extent applicable to compilations of such works.

Independent verification should be sought for any data, advice or recommendations contained in this book. In addition, no responsibility is assumed by the Publisher for any injury and/or damage to persons or property arising from any methods, products, instructions, ideas or otherwise contained in this publication.

This publication is designed to provide accurate and authoritative information with regard to the subject matter covered herein. It is sold with the clear understanding that the Publisher is not engaged in rendering legal or any other professional services. If legal or any other expert assistance is required, the services of a competent person should be sought. FROM A DECLARATION OF PARTICIPANTS JOINTLY ADOPTED BY A COMMITTEE OF THE AMERICAN BAR ASSOCIATION AND A COMMITTEE OF PUBLISHERS.

Additional color graphics may be available in the e-book version of this book.

Library of Congress Cataloging-in-Publication Data

ISBN: 978-1-53617-061-0

Published by Nova Science Publishers, Inc. † New York

Contents

Preface vii

Chapter 1 The Breastfeeding Relationship, Child Development and Maternal Health 1
Mary Rheeston

Chapter 2 Breast Milk for Premature Infants: Nutritive and Health Aspects 27
Nikoleta M. Lugonja and Snežana D. Spasić

Chapter 3 Breastfeeding, Use of Common Substances and Offspring's Weight Gain and Growth during Infancy and Childhood 69
Edmond D. Shenassa, Fiona M. Jardine and Anne Lise Brantsæter

Chapter 4 Lessons from the Past: How Research, Programs and Legislation Impacted Infant and Young Child Nutrition from Prehistory to the End of the 19th Century 103
Veronika Scherbaum and Elizabeth Hormann

Chapter 5	Use of Breast Milk and Breastfeeding as a Non Pharmacological Method for Procedural Pain Management *Ayşe Şener Taplak and Sevinç Polat*	141
Chapter 6	Long-Term Impacts of Breastfeeding on Prevention of Non-Communicable Diseases *Motahar Heidari-Beni and Roya Kelishadi*	179
Index		197
Related Nova Publications		205

PREFACE

This compilation opens by exploring how the physical and psychological elements of breastfeeding are intrinsically linked to a child's development and the mother's wellbeing, both in the short and long terms. Babies who are exclusively breastfed see advantages in cognitive and language development, as well as protection against disease.

The authors assess the main nutritive factors of breast milk, the use of fortifier as breast milk supplement, the significance of microelements in preterm nutrition, and health outcomes related to breast milk for preterm infants.

The current knowledge on substance exposure through breastfeeding is also addressed, specifically how it may influence weight gain and growth during infancy and childhood, and whether the timing of that exposure may alter those outcomes.

Recommendations and common feeding practices are closely linked with political and socio-economic conditions of different time periods and are embedded in culture-specific strategies for food, nutrition security and health care. As such, a review of the events and developments in the area of infant and young child nutrition, programming and human rights issues from prehistory until the end of the 19th century is provided.

The penultimate study is aimed to provide an updated synthesis of the current evidence for the effectiveness of breastfeeding and breast milk feeding in the reduction of procedural pain in preterm and full-term born infants.

Non-communicable diseases are usually caused by interaction of genetic factors, gender, age, ethnicity, environmental exposures, and lifestyle behaviors. Primary should start with an emphasis on improving breastfeeding practices. Consequently, the closing chapter aims to summarize the current literature on the long-term effects of breastfeeding on the prevention of non-communicable diseases.

Chapter 1 - The body of evidence exploring the effect of breastfeeding on child development and maternal health is overwhelmingly positive. Key themes emerge from the research reinforcing the World Health Organisation's recommendations of exclusive breastfeeding for six months onwards. Physical and psychological elements of breastfeeding are intrinsically linked for optimal impact on a child's development and the mother's wellbeing both in the short and long term. Cognitive and language development and protection against disease show advantages for babies who are exclusively breastfed. In addition to the physiological components of breastmilk, maternal sensitivity within their relationship is an important feature of nurturing a child's development. Providing emotional support to pregnant women and breastfeeding mothers supports responsive breastfeeding and maternal health.

Chapter 2 - Breast milk is considered to be the only and the best nutrition for newborn infants until six months of age. However, some of the most important problems regarding the nutrition of infants after preterm delivery are due to the fact that preterm milk is produced before complete maturation of mammary glands and that the preterm infant's gastrointestinal tract is not mature enough at the time of partition. Since human milk has unique properties in promoting gastrointestinal maturation and immunological benefits, it is very important to implement strategies of fortification to appropriately actuate its benefits. Donor breast milk from milk banks is widely used when mother's own milk is not available or when it is in short supply for preterm infants. While donor breast milk retains some of the biological properties and clinical benefits of mother's own milk, it requires additional care in terms of fortification, especially if the donor milk is from a pool of term breast milk which is somewhat different than preterm breast milk.

As nutritional strategies improve, the ultimate goal is to minimize extrauterine growth restriction and promote appropriate growth and development of premature infants. Another problem with breast milk, which is quite often overlooked, is that after six months, there is not enough of essential microelements (Zn, Fe and Cu) to satisfy baby's needs, and therefore, the milk must be effectively supplemented.

In this chapter the authors review the following aspects of breast milk for preterm infants: 1) The main nutritive factors of breast milk; 2) The use of fortifier as breast milk supplement; 3) Significance of microelements in preterm nutrition; and 4) Health outcomes of breast milk for preterm infants.

Chapter 3 - Among the most important benefits of breastfeeding is the optimal weight gain and growth during infancy that is experienced by infants who are exclusively breastfed for the first six months of life. Appropriate weight gain during infancy is among the most important determinants of healthy development. Infancy weight gain, but not necessarily weight gain during early childhood, has been consistently linked with obesity over the lifecourse. Approximately 20% of the risk for becoming overweight during childhood and 30% of the risk for obesity during adulthood is attributable to weight gain during infancy. Because obesity can become intransigent during early childhood, obesogenic processes are best disrupted during pregnancy and infancy, a time of plasticity in neural communication between adipocytes in the brain and other organs and a window of time when the parents are most amenable to changing their behaviors.

Influences on infancy weight gain act synergistically and the timing of exposure to these other influences is important. Among the most prevalent influences on infancy weight gain are maternal smoking as well as caffeine intake during and after pregnancy. Direct and secondhand exposure to cannabis is another influence that is gaining in prevalence.

Unfortunately, antismoking programs are of limited availability and have high relapse rates. For this and other related reasons, maternal and paternal smoking during and immediately after pregnancy remains highly prevalent globally. Caffeine intake is similarly prevalent due to its social acceptability and ubiquity. Although cannabis use is not yet as widespread as these other substances, its use is increasing due to its rise in popularity and growing legality. While the authors have a reasonably good understanding of the effects of smoking and caffeine intake during and after pregnancy, the authors' understanding of their interactions with breastfeeding and their timing remains rudimentary at best. The authors' understanding of effects of cannabis exposure is even more limited, but enough research now exists to draw preliminary conclusions. A better understanding of how these determinants may interact with breastfeeding to influence weight gain and growth during infancy and childhood can inform interventions to promote optimum infant development.

Current knowledge on each substance will be discussed in terms of prevalence and sources of intake, bioavailability, exposure through breastfeeding and how that may influence weight gain and growth during infancy and childhood, and whether the timing of that exposure may alter those outcomes.

Chapter 4 - Recommendations and common feeding practices are closely linked with political and socio-economic conditions of different time periods and are embedded in culture-specific strategies for food, nutrition security and health care.

This narrative review addresses events and developments in the area of infant and young child nutrition as well as related research, programming and human rights issues from prehistory until the end of the 19th century. It also aims to draw key lessons from past findings and evolutions which took place in many societies and are highly relevant in today's context.

While artificial infant feeding has been always an important causal factor of child mortality, since middle of the 19th Century, environmental improvements and pasteurization of cow's milk have contributed to declining death rates. In addition, proper care and nutrition of young children with respect to health, growth and development as well as the essential role of a close mother-infant-relationship have been increasingly recognized. However, many socio-economic, cultural and legal constraints to support and protect adequate infant and young child feeding also play an important role.

Chapter 5 - Newborns and infants require needle-related painful procedures for scheduled childhood immunizations, as well as medical procedures performed for diagnostic and treatment purposes during the course of childhood illnesses. Uncontrolled pain causes clinical instability as a result of development of complications such as changes in heart rate, respiratory rate, blood pressure, intracranial pressure, oxygen saturation along with intraventricular hemorrhaging. Recurrent pain experienced for the purpose of diagnosis and treatment leads to atrophy in the brain of the infant, which can result in neurodevelopmental problems and a decrease in the subcortical white and gray matter in the brain.

The prevention or minimization of pain is the right of any newborns and infants. As infants experience a healthy neonatal period when their pain is under control, their duration of stay in hospital is reduced and their growth and development can accelerate, which contributes positively to the national economy. However, studies on pain in infants reveal that 40-60% of infants do not receive any preventive or therapeutic application during painful procedures. In recognizing the adverse consequences of untreated pain in infants, national guidelines for evidence informed pain assessment and management practices have been developed. An intervention recommended in such guidelines for procedural pain management is breastmilk and breastfeeding.

This study is aimed to provide an updated synthesis of the current state of the evidence for the effectiveness of breastfeeding and breast milk feeding in reducing procedural pain in preterm and full-term born infants. A systematic search of key electronic databases (PubMed, Science Direct, Google Scholar) will be sought. The main criteria are behavioral or physiological indicators and compound pain scores and other clinically important results reported by the authors.

The findings of the studies show that breastfeeding is more effective in reducing pain during painful interventions such as heel lance, aspiration and vaccination in newborns and infants, compared to studies using breast milk or breast milk smell alone.

Chapter 6 - Current evidence reported that non-communicable diseases (NCDs) including cardiovascular diseases, cancers, chronic respiratory diseases, and diabetes originate from early life. NCDs are usually caused by interaction of genetic factors, gender, age, ethnicity, environmental exposures, and lifestyle behaviors.

Breastfeeding is perfectly designed for the child's nutritional needs and it is the most advantageous feeding option for infants. In addition to its short-term benefits, it has several beneficial effects for prevention of NCDs for both mothers and children. Breast milk provides all the energy and nutrients that infants need for the first six months of life and is critical for sustaining the health of newborns and infants. Despite the beneficial effects of breastfeeding, it is still below the World Health Organization (WHO) recommendation in many countries.

Many studies showed long-term protective effects of adequate breastfeeding during infancy on NCDs particularly on hypertension, obesity, diabetes, dyslipidemia, and cardiovascular diseases at individual and population levels. However, there are controversial findings about these effects. Recall bias for exclusivity and duration of breastfeeding and low availability of infant nutrition data in retrospective cohorts may lead to inconsistent results between studies.

The primordial prevention of NCDs should start with an emphasis on improving breastfeeding practices. This chapter aims to summarize the current literature on the long-term effects of breastfeeding on prevention of NCDs and their risk factors.

In: New Research on Breastfeeding ...
Editor: Kai Santos Melo

ISBN: 978-1-53617-061-0
© 2020 Nova Science Publishers, Inc.

Chapter 1

THE BREASTFEEDING RELATIONSHIP, CHILD DEVELOPMENT AND MATERNAL HEALTH

Mary Rheeston[*]
Solihull, UK

ABSTRACT

The body of evidence exploring the effect of breastfeeding on child development and maternal health is overwhelmingly positive. Key themes emerge from the research reinforcing the World Health Organisation's recommendations of exclusive breastfeeding for six months onwards. Physical and psychological elements of breastfeeding are intrinsically linked for optimal impact on a child's development and the mother's wellbeing both in the short and long term. Cognitive and language development and protection against disease show advantages for babies who are exclusively breastfed. In addition to the physiological components of breastmilk, maternal sensitivity within their relationship is

---

[*] Corresponding Author's E-mail: mary.rheeston@heartofengland.nhs.uk.

an important feature of nurturing a child's development. Providing emotional support to pregnant women and breastfeeding mothers supports responsive breastfeeding and maternal health.

Imagine you leave the safety of the womb to enter a world where your continued survival is dependent on being taken care of, receiving adequate nutrition, fulfilling your growth and development potential, protection against infection, developing relationships and the physical and emotional health of your primary caregiver. Where do you source such particulates of life? Well there is a confident body of evidence indicating that the process probably begins before you were conceived and definitely while you were in the womb. Nature has put a considerable amount of effort into its design of the fundamental structures to protect you. One of the key building blocks with the potential to affect how stable your future health and development will be is that your mother is able to breastfeed you with milk produced by her own body. In doing so she will give you the necessary nutrients and protection you need for life while at the same time enhancing her own wellbeing. Basic chemical and emotional pathways will have been secured prenatally and many other synapses and systems are ready to connect after you are born. In addition the action of breastfeeding will invite you to experience intricate layers of human relationships the origins of which in later life will be forgotten. It is possible to acquire these elements from alternative means but it is being cared for and breastfed by your mother in optimal circumstances that will provide you with the best advantage for a healthy, happy and productive life.

The World Health Organisation identifies early child development as a priority area of work highlighting that an estimated 250 million children or 43 percent of children in low and middle income countries do not reach their full potential. Their document Nurturing Care classifies early childhood development as between the ages of 0-8 years encompassing physical, social, emotional, cognitive and motor development. The report describes adequate nutrition as a key component in supporting children to reach their full potential and states that 'young children flourish on exclusive breastfeeding' with a strong emphasis that the way in which breastmilk is offered should contribute to positive social and emotional interactions between mother and child [1].

This growing integration of thinking and evidence between physical and psychological elements of nurturing a child includes breastfeeding. Each discipline working in the field of child development and maternal health understandably focuses on overcoming individual deficits in their areas of work. The emerging blend of neuroscience with psychology, with its impact on child development and health outcomes over the last three decades, has prompted researchers to increase efforts to connect these different areas of research. This is important if the evidence is to guide us towards overcoming localised and global difficulties. Human development is after all multidimensional and if we are to strive to improve outcomes for a child's health and development it should be recognised that children are not limited to the findings of each independent field. A 'child is the holistic synthesis of all these domains' and so should be the synthesis of our ideas and curiosity [2]. A literature search with the intention of exploring elements of breastfeeding and cognitive development will present the reader with articles examining genetic factors, IQ measurements with possible differences in results for full term and preterm babies, milk components, neurodevelopment, confounders such as maternal intelligence, short term developmental gains and long term outcomes, effects of breastfeeding duration, 'skin to skin' immediately after birth, maternal sensitivity, confidence and mental health and parenting behaviours and perhaps most recently epigenetics. Making sense of the research and their relationship to one another can be challenging. However many who are working to improve health outcomes for children have a determined perspective that breastfeeding has more to offer than just a feeding function. Consequently, innovative studies, programmes and interventions exist and aim to bring about real change in the lives of mothers, babies and families. But more about that later, for now we will explore what the evidence base says about the effect of breastfeeding on child development and maternal health.

The volume of research on the subject of breastfeeding is broad and complex and has accelerated in the past 50 years. When scrolling through the plethora of studies it is easy to become distracted in the subject matter investigating breastfeeding. Both child development and maternal health have been extensively researched and written about. It might be expected that with decades of data at our disposal the search to understand the effect and role of breastfeeding on mother and infant would be concluded. However, in some areas the debate continues as to the exact nature of its impact especially for emotional development. Research is perhaps clearest when discussing the role of breastfeeding in reducing infant mortality and morbidity rates for common infectious diseases causing diarrhoea and vomiting [3]. In 1984 Freachem and Koblinsky's review exploring interventions to control diarrhoeal diseases through the promotion of breastfeeding suggested that theoretical calculations based on reviewed data could lead to a reduction of mortality rates of babies dying from diarrheal disease by 24-27%. When comparing non breastfed babies to those exclusively breastfed the mortality risk was 25 times greater for non-breastfed infants [4]. Their work recognised the importance of exclusive breastfeeding in the first six months of life and contributed to the current recommendation by the World Health Organisation and UNICEF that infants should be exclusively breastfed until they are six months of age. The powerful immunological components of breastmilk together with its nutritional value of satisfying the growth needs of the infant have further informed public health organisations, leading to recommendations that breastfeeding should be continued alongside responsive complementary feeding for the first two years [5].

    Breastfeeding has also been associated with protecting babies from sudden infant death syndrome, a highly emotive topic that understandably remains prominent in the consciousness of parents and professionals. The exact mechanism of links between breastfeeding and babies dying in this way are still not completely understood. However, the source of protection may be related to the findings that breastfeeding infants are more easily roused from sleep and have an immunological advantage that supports their immature immune system [6]. Moving on from the first year of life an association has been shown between breastfeeding and a reduced risk of developing asthma and allergies as well as lower levels of obesity in childhood, adolescence and adults [7, 8]. These areas of research have significant public health implications for personal health, whole population trends and economic consequences. Breastfeeding does not offer 100% protection against disease, but it can provide the infant with sufficient defences and opportunities to protect them. Indirectly, it also contributes to supporting child development and maternal mental health. Short infrequent episodes of illness where recovery is reasonably quick probably have little impact on a child's overall development. This is where breastfeeding and the efficiency of the immune system are so impressive. The mother's body when exposed to the same pathogens as the infant, will manufacture a customised immunological response and deliver this to the baby in regular doses through her breastmilk. When ill the infant will more than likely seek comfort from increased suckling and quieten with close proximity to the mother. The increase in the number of breastfeeds will in turn pass more antibodies to the baby in the breastmilk. It will also soothe the baby and trigger the release of oxytocin in the mother's brain with each feed creating a calming influence on the mother's level of anxiety. When her infant is ill of course she may still be anxious but with the benefit of the anti-stress properties of that accompany breastfeeding she may feel more able to manage both herself and the needs of her baby [9].

Child development is generally accepted as the sequence of predictable changes that occur during the period from infancy to adolescent. Their order is largely genetically controlled with environmental influences affecting the speed, quality and potential of their progress. Individuals may not follow the exact order as others however there are agreed areas of development that apply to all children. These include physical, cognitive, emotional, and motor development. The stages of child development often referred to as milestones moves rapidly in the early weeks and months. Developmental progress is screened and examined by parents and professionals intensive in the first year of life and a baby's progress can be both a source of reassurance and considerable anxiety for parents.

A child's cognitive development and its association with breastfeeding is an area of particular interest to researchers. Cognitive development incorporates the processing of information, memory, social skills, language development, logical reasoning, planning, and problem solving. Breastmilk is known to contain components that are essential for early brain and retinal development. Docosahexaenoic acid (DHA) and arachidonic acid (AA) the most abundant polysaturated fatty acids have been identified as crucial to support brain growth [10]. Studies investigating association between breastfeeding and cognitive development have suggested neurological functioning relies on adequate levels of these fatty acids. Their role in accelerating growth in a baby's young brain, central nervous system and retinal development is vital and preterm babies who have reduced fat stores at birth and are particularly vulnerable. Unlike the full term baby they will not have had the opportunity in the third trimester of fetal accretion of DHA [11].

Two notable meta-analysis in the last twenty years have reviewed studies investigating breastfeeding and cognitive development. Anderson et al's 1999 review provided important data by observing differences between cognitive function of babies who were breastfed and formula fed. Twenty studies were reviewed and the authors concluded that babies who were breastfed had a 3.2-point advantage in their cognitive development over infants who were formula fed. Their higher score remained after adjustment for 15 key cofactors that included duration of breastfeeding, race or ethnicity, sex, and maternal smoking history, age, intelligence, education, training and paternal education. It is also significant that their review suggested that not only was a baby's cognitive development impacted early by breastfeeding its effect was sustained through to adolescence. In addition the meta-analysis identified benefits for low birth babies' cognitive development were even greater. The results were almost double at 5.18 points ($P < 0.001$) compared with full term breastfed infants whose advantage was 2.66 points over the formula fed infants [12]. Together with these findings they highlighted the effect breastfeeding duration had on cognitive development, a theme that has permeated many other aspects of breastfeeding. Several studies recorded incremental benefits from six months onwards a finding that is compatible with the current recommendation that babies should be exclusively breastfed for the first six months.

The second meta-analysis published in 2015 examined the association between breastfeeding and intelligence. Results showed an improved performance in intelligence tests of breastfed infants of 3.44 points and as with the Anderson et al. review the positive effect on cognitive function was maintained in childhood and adolescence. Increased confidence in adjusting for confounders has emerged in the intervening years between the two meta-analyses, especially relevant to maternal intelligence. The 2015 systematic review revealed that studies controlling for maternal IQ demonstrated pooled odds ratio: 2.62 (95% confidence interval: 1.25; 3.98) [13]. As part of the systematic review the authors highlighted the findings of a cluster randomised study by Kramer et al. where intelligence quotient showed a remarkable mean difference of +7.5 in favour of breastfeeding. Not all studies reported supported the higher cognitive measures for breastfeeding [14].

Both meta-analyses acknowledged that the association between breastfeeding and cognitive development is not completely positive and a small number of studies when adjusted for confounders showed no increase in cognitive function in favour of breastfeeding. A study of approximately 8000 participants that investigated the cognitive and non cognitive development of 3 to 5 year olds enrolled in Growing Up in Ireland were surprised by the findings showing no statistically significance gain for cognitive abilities and expressive vocabulary for children who had been breastfed as an infant. In addition to measuring cognitive development and language, the researchers included the Strengths and Difficulties Questionnaire to assess child behaviour problems [15]. Interestingly this was the one positive result found in the study. Children who were fully breastfed for six months or more had slightly lower parent-rated hyperactivity at 3 years that remained statistically significant after adjustment. Association or causal effects relating to skin to skin or nutritional content of breastmilk were considered but data was unavailable to explore connections so the authors could only recommend future studies to examine behavioural outcomes [16]. This finding is important as it links breastfeeding to maternal sensitivity and the development of self-regulation in the child development. Our capacity to learn and develop requires us to be able to pay attention and regulate our emotional state and behaviour. At the age of 3 years these abilities may be a more important measure.

Having a score identifying a child's IQ has been a popular way of comparing a child's cognitive development and parents and professionals have been encouraged by the presentation of evidence stating that it is higher for breastfeeding infants than that of those who have been formula fed. While the data is accurate, overall findings confirm that infants who are breastfed show higher IQ scores, it also the case that in evolutionary terms human breastfeeding behaviour is the norm. So perhaps by describing it in this way we miss the obvious: that really it should be considered as the baseline measurement and that babies who are formula fed would naturally therefore be in a deficit for cognitive development. In today's society conversations around breastfeeding and formula feeding can be extremely sensitive and it is understandable that the way in which we communicate this information to parents needs to be carried out with thoughtfulness and care. Some scientists who view breastfeeding as the norm have suggested that lower cognitive scores should therefore be considered abnormal [17].

A child's cognitive capacity is an aspect of child development that is of significant importance to parents. Although when breastfeeding her baby a mother is probably not thinking about the scientific findings of population studies she may be receptive to the knowledge that her choice to breastfeed her baby may add to their intellectual growth and development. Kramer et al. (ibid) made a relevant point in relation to parents, breastfeeding and cognitive development in their discussion. They refer to research that suggests that breastfeeding mothers are more likely to provide a stimulating environment and breastfeeding may be a marker linking to parenting practice [18, 19]. They also suggest that there may be subtle differences in the interactions of breastfeeding mothers with their babies that are difficult to measure.

Biological factors are generally accepted as playing a role and in particular DHA and AA, two of the most prominent fatty acids. Their levels reach peak disposition in the last trimester of pregnancy and first year of life coinciding with rapid neural growth in the baby's brain that incorporates pathways for cognitive and language development. Breastfeeding is an intimate act between the mother and infant where both are attempting to adjust to each other so that the mother can produce milk for her baby and the baby is able to receive breast milk. Breastfeeding is an important step at the beginning of a child's development. It is also one of the earliest experiences of parenting that will in turn influence later parenting practices that may influence a child's development. How a parent understands and interprets the cues their infant, communicates with them and the way in which they respond may have its foundations in the moments of interaction as the mother offers her baby the breast. How a parent encourages the baby to search for the breast or soothes them so they are able to coordinate their body and mouth towards the nipple may be witnessed later in more sophisticated demonstrations of their parenting style.

Parents are extremely influential in supporting and nurturing their infant's language development. Parenting, breastfeeding and language development are bound together as parents help and encourage their baby as they navigate the complex elements of language acquisition. We all know that language development is not just all about the phonics and sentence construction or avoiding double negatives. Communication is complex and it is most noticeable when it does not go smoothly.

The evidence base linking breastfeeding and language development exists and as with cognitive development, breastfed infants on balance show an advantage over formula fed babies. The range and volume of studies specifically targeting language development cannot compete with the numbers solely investigating breastfeeding's association to cognitive development. Language often appears in studies investigating cognitive and motor development, which is not surprising as they are the areas of child development that are generally most noticeable. A study in Greece of 540 mother-child pairs showed longer duration of breastfeeding exceeding 6 months was associated with higher receptive communication that persisted after adjustment of identified confounders [20]. The study also found increased scores for motor and cognitive development associated with breastfeeding for more than 6 months. However, the evidence base examining the influences of breastfeeding on a child's motor development are more mixed, with other studies suggesting little or no impact on motor development [21]. A large cross-sectional data set of 22,399 children in the United States was examined from the 2003 National Survey of Children's Health. Mothers were asked questions relating to their level of concern about their child's development that included expressive and receptive language development. The mean age of the sample was 2.79 years and breastfeeding data was acquired from the mother's recall. Although there were adjustments for some confounders it was not possible to do so for mother's IQ as this was not available to the researchers. Breastfeeding mothers expressed fewer concerns about their children's language development. The decrease was evident for mothers who breastfed their infants for 3months or more and levels of concern continued to reduce in mothers who breastfed for 9 months or more [22]. Other studies have also suggested lactation duration can be an influencing factor in promoting language development. 604 children under the age of 3 years were selected by a three-stage stratified random sample from the Balochistan – Early Childhood Development Project in Pakistan. The results of an adjusted and unadjusted analysis showed children who were breastfed from more than 12 months had a language and cognitive advantage. In addition data was collected for immunisation and this showed children who had received the full immunisation schedule compared to children who were not immunised were 2.91 times more likely to demonstrate age appropriate language development. Not being protected from disease with the risk of experiencing episodes of ill health can deprive an infant of valuable time for all aspects of development and language development is one such area. In addition being breastfed affords the infant the extra protection of the immunological benefits of breastmilk [23]. Each study has its own unique feature, but what is consistent are the results that place breastfeeding at the forefront for a child achieves the best outcomes for their development.

From these studies and many others it is possible to conclude that breastfeeding can positively impact on a child's language development. The evidence base for just how this occurs is less precise. Breastfeeding is not alone in its function. Genes, physiology and psychology are intricately woven together through breastfeeding to allow the infant to enter the social world of communication. Nature and nurture coexist as the two worlds working together to ensure that the quality of positive early child development is sustained into adulthood. This is why studies indicating that breastfeeding mothers have an increased sensitivity to the needs of their baby should be afforded equal status to those showing advantages to IQ and the nutritional value of breastmilk.

In the moments immediately after birth skin to skin contact is championed as a way to encouraging bonding and promoting breastfeeding activity. The practice of laying the baby against the mother's bare chest aims to initiate instinctive behaviours in the mother and baby and stimulate biological responses [24]. Skin to skin contact has a calming effect on each of their nervous systems and areas of the brain vital for regulating their physiological and psychological states. In the mother's body the physical skin to skin contact enhances the release of oxytocin providing a boost to the process of bonding and attachment. It is the beginning of their relationship outside the womb that under the right circumstances is filled with hope and expectation. If a mother continues to breastfeed the practicalities of breastfeeding mean that skin to skin contact occurs more frequently than with bottle feeding. In the womb babies are known to react to the rhythm of their mother's voice and as they are laid on her chest post birth they open their eyes to search for the face that matches the voice they heard in the womb [25]. By no coincidence the distance between the breast and the mothers face is approximately the same as the newborn's visual range, approximately 20-25 cm or 8-10 inches. Immediately after birth the infant combines these essential pieces of information to identify the person they expect to feed and nurture them.

Being breastfed by their mother means that in the early days and months of life a baby is able to concentrate on learning a single language of interaction with one main carer through the feeding relationship before accommodating a wider scope of interactions and relationships with others. One of the challenges for the newborn when being bottle feeding is that they are often fed by several adults and although this can be helpful for bonding with the other parent and close family members for example, one wonders what are the implications for the baby's development. Many adults who have fed a baby will tell you that there is something intensely satisfying about feeding a baby and hearing the reassuring burp as they are winded feels like a shared triumph. Our desire to feed a baby is probably in our genes. However, from the baby's perspective in the very early days and months, perhaps we should ask, is it in the interests of the baby to be fed by more than one person and what are the implications for their development? It is clear that babies can adapt and if hungry will take milk that is offered, but knowing what we now know about children's emotional and cognitive development might it be in the baby's interests for the feeding relationship to be protected? This could be a controversial idea and it would not suggest that the father or partner caring for the baby should be excluded from the feeding experience if formula milk via a bottle is the chosen mode of feeding. There are advantages for the father or partner feeding the baby that can facilitate bonding. This is more enhanced if feeding is carried out in a responsive way as recommended by Unicef in their Infant formula and responsive feeding leaflet [26]. Unicef point out that true responsive feeding is not possible with bottle feeding but that supporting parents who give most of the feeds in the early weeks of life can help build a secure relationship [27]. Having a conversation that begins in the antenatal period between the parents and with professionals about what feeding means for everyone should become the norm so that the impact of the feeding experience can be optimised for the infant.

The sensitivity of the mother's ongoing interactions with her baby is pivotal in how she communicates and adapts her responses whether feeding or engaging in other interactions. Her deep and often unconscious knowledge of her baby can be crucial as the baby transitions from one stage of development the next. Breastfeeding mothers have been shown to have increased sensitivity to their babies and once again breastfeeding duration appears to be a notable factor [28, 29]. A systematic review of studies investigating associations between breastfeeding and maternal responsiveness confirmed an association exists for increased sensitivity of breastfeeding mothers. Despite reviewing over 40 studies dating back to

1970 the reviewers were still left wondering how and why maternal responsiveness was consistently shown to be associated with breastfeeding. One hypothesis proposed is that breastfeeding mothers have to exert more energy into trusting their baby to self-regulate their feeding requirement and tailor their breastfeed behaviours to the baby's cues that indicate they are satisfied [30]. Bottle feeding mothers on the other hand have a greater ability to assess and control how much formula milk their infant was drinking. This is an interesting perspective and is not unfamiliar to my own observations when working as a Health Visitor in the United Kingdom. My experience was that in very broad terms breastfeeding mothers worried that their babies were not taking enough breastmilk and would anxiously watch their baby for signs they were satisfied or still hungry. Whereas bottle feeding mothers worried their babies were drinking too much milk while at the same time anxiously encouraging the baby to finish the bottle. Both mothers exhibited signs of anxiety, but for different reasons and consequently on reflection their feeding relationship with their baby also differed. Breastfeeding mothers checked their babies more often whereas bottle feeding mothers checked the bottle. Of course this is anecdotal and there were degrees of sensitivity and responsiveness for both feeding mother and infant dyads but my sense was that there was a distinction that resonates with the research findings of many studies.

Responsiveness has become the zeitgeist of relationships in current times. It would be wrong to suggest that the focus on maternal sensitivity is a new phenomenon. As with many theories and trends the understandings we have today are the result of many years of mindful innovators, enlightened researchers and courageous practitioners. We have them to thank for their willingness to reframe what they previously believed to be a firm truth and push forward with a new paradigm. As we wonder what underpins the breastfeeding mother's capacity to be responsive to her infant with sensitivity that makes a difference to her infant's future emotional and developmental progress, we might consider professionals whose work has added to our understanding. Brazelton and his colleagues began their research in the late 1960s that was later published in 1974 [31]. Brazelton had a particular interest in early mother-child interactions and through his research he presented his scientific findings to colleagues and the wider professional community with a fresh appreciation of the sophisticated nature of interactions between the mother and baby. Brazelton used the term reciprocity to describe interactions he observed and compared them to a sequence of steps akin to a 'dance'. This simple set of steps is considered to be one of the basic building blocks of not only how we communicate but also of how we regulate ourselves and is fundamental to the development of relationships [32]. Turn taking behaviours develop as the baby sucks and rests during a feed giving rise to the beginnings of a conversation. Turn taking is fundamental for communication and language development [33]. Observing a breastfeeding mother and infant interacting in ordinary everyday events, it can appear as though nothing spectacular is taking place. What goes unnoticed or unseen are the biochemical, hormonal and psychosocial exchanges that occur alongside the subtle second by second verbal and non verbal interactions as both mother and baby adjust to one another [34]. Paired with the finding that breastfeeding mothers show increased sensitivity in their interactions with their infant it makes sense that there may well be later advantages in language development for babies who are breastfed. One of the most startling discoveries in Brazelton's research was that both the infant and mother were active in the process. The mother alone did not regulate the interactions, instead the baby was an equal partner. Having a mother who facilitators your developing sense of agency and confidence as you explore your interactions with the world is just as important as having access to a stimulating environment to move your development forward.

Douglas also suggests that reciprocity is the basis for the development of language and communication and went further to indicate that it is instrumental in the development of the patterns and rhythms we establish for eating, drinking, waking, sleeping, self-control and regulation [35]. Her work has led to the development of a theoretical model integrating the concept of reciprocity together with two other well established concepts containment and behaviour management. The concepts are used as a way of thinking in a wide range of applications across the spectrum of emotional wellbeing and parenting. The approach that has been developed recognises how important the mother's emotional availability and capacity to think is for her to be able to tune into her infant's needs. For all mothers emotional support is important when feeding their babies and for mothers who are breastfeeding or who are thinking of breastfeeding their baby it is especially relevant if breastfeeding rates are to increase more rapidly. There has been progress in recent decades but it has been slow and the disparity even amongst developed countries is startling. In the UK for example breastfeeding rates have been recorded as low as 44% in a report by Public Health England 2016/17 compared with impressive breastfeeding rates of 71% in Norway [36].

Mothers and professionals have had access to the knowledge that breastfeeding is good for babies and offers protection for breastfeeding women against diseases such as breast cancer for years. As with many of the benefits to the infant, published meta analyses suggest that there may be an impact on breast cancer risk in the mother linked to the length of time a mother breastfeeds her infant [37, 38]. A review that included 13 studies for breast cancer showed a 2% increase in protection per five month period of breastfeeding duration. However the same review found other studies, albeit fewer in number, reporting no significant association between breastfeeding duration and reduces risk of breast cancer [39]. Other health benefits aligned with breastfeeding include reduced risks of ovarian cancer and type 2 diabetes [40, 41]. Interestingly these studies also showed an effect that could be related to the duration of breastfeeding. The risk of ovarian cancer was reduced when a woman breastfed for as little as 3 months and there was a strong graded association for type 2 diabetes increasing from a reduced risk of 25% up to six months lactation, rising to 47% for six months or more.

These physical health outcomes for mothers are interesting and as I said earlier it is easy to become distracted by the wealth of knowledge at our finger tips. So let us return to the question 'how do we increase the number of women who will make the choice to breastfeed their baby?' Programmes solely offering information to mothers and families are beneficial. However, the experience of becoming a parent can be a very emotional experience and overwhelming emotions can be troublesome.

They can disrupt our thinking and ability to make use of this valuable knowledge. Programmes that are relationship based in design are more likely to address such issues as feelings. In Northern Ireland for example, the Early Intervention Transformation Programme (EITP) has brought together six government agencies together with Atlantic Philanthropies. It aims to equip parents with skills to give their children the best start in life and reduce the risk of poor outcomes later in life. The Social Change Initiative starts in the antenatal period, training 350 midwives in the Solihull Approach that supports one to one work and groups of parents. The six week antenatal parenting group includes both practical aspects of labour and birth as well as a focus on the feeding relationship and the emerging relationship between the baby and parent [42]. Data collection is ongoing. However preliminary results as yet unpublished have shown that in the antenatal period 90% of parents have become more confident about what to expect, coping with labour and birth and becoming a parent [43]. The programme is offered to first time mothers showed that 75% of parents who attended the programme attempted to breastfeed and 60% were still breastfeeding on discharge from hospital after giving birth. This is in comparison with 47% of all mothers in Northern Ireland [44]. Achieving significant change is challenging and by developing a strategy that is built on collaboration, evidence base and scale, Northern Ireland are seeing the beginnings of an encouraging increase in breastfeeding rates in a relatively short period of time.

If targets indicated by UNICEF for exclusive breastfeeding during the 6 months are to be achieved support for breastfeeding mothers is extremely important. The quality and type of support provided for breastfeeding mothers has required thought and planning. Previous to the current directions by the Baby Friendly Initiative, few programmes could demonstrate a reliable evidence base. Many were run by enthusiastic practitioners, but lacked consistency and were reliant on short term funding. One form of support that has become increasingly integrated into programmes, is popular and shows a promise as an effective mode of support is the role of the peer breastfeeding supporter. Mothers who have breastfed themselves have a unique perspective and with appropriate training and supervision add strength to initiatives for parents in the antenatal and postnatal periods. In areas where breastfeeding rates are low, peer breastfeeding supporters can often access and develop trusting relationships within a community that professional input alone can struggle to achieve. The evidence base is improving and a systematic review and meta-analysis in 2017 by Shakya et al. concluded that community-based peer support was effective in increasing exclusive breastfeeding in both high, and low and medium income countries, but more so in the latter [45]. Interestingly the reasons did not relate to the peer supporter rather social preferences for formula feeding in high income countries and less favourable attitudes and high cost of formula in low and middle income countries. These findings demonstrate that peer breastfeeding support is beneficial but once again the question that arises is why and how they are effective. Other studies that have explored this dynamic suggest it is in the quality of relationship between the mother and peer supporter. Developing a mutually supportive relationship is central to supporting the emotions that mothers may experience when breastfeeding [46]. An evaluation that interviewed mothers attending community breastfeeding groups where peer supporters' training was underpinned by a robust theoretical relationship based model reported feeding emotionally supported and empowered They described breastfeeding environment as their first experience where breastfeeding was the norm and ' For once, we are in the majority.' They felt as ease and accepted even if they were feeling down or upset [47]. A separate study explored the peer breastfeeding supporters' experience of using the Solihull Approach model in their peer supporter role. They found the training and its application in their role had increased their confidence, creating positive feelings and enabled them to detect their own stressors. When interviewed the peer supporters described witnessing reciprocity in action when observing a mother and baby interacting through breastfeeding [48].

The body of evidence exploring the effect of breastfeeding on child development and maternal health is overwhelmingly positive. Nutrition may be the most obvious purpose of breastmilk however breastfeeding has a labyrinth of interconnected functions that have the potential to secure a healthy life trajectory for the infant and maintain wellbeing in the mother. Many of these functions are embedded in the relationship between the mother and baby and as a consequence it is difficult to talk about one without the other. Cognitive development does not develop in isolation. There are biological components in breastmilk for neurodevelopment that work alongside a mother's sensitivity towards her baby. Providing a stimulating socio emotional and physical environment for optimum development will in part be influenced by the breastfeeding experience. The same is relevant for language development and emotional development, not to mention the calming effect that oxytocin can have on the mother's mental health while also helping her bond with her baby.

Key themes emerge in the research investigating breastfeeding, child development and maternal health. One of the most prominent findings is the significance of breastfeeding duration on outcomes. In line with the World Health Organisation's recommendation of exclusive breastfeeding many studies report better outcomes when babies are fed for six months onwards achieve high scores in a variety of measures.

In addition to the decades of research that supports breastfeeding as the best method of feeding babies, evidence from the field of epigenetics is beginning to increase our understanding of the mechanisms of both short and long term health outcomes for mother and child. Epigenetics has been studied since the 1940's and is the term used to describe to explain changes in gene expression and inherited expression states that are passed from parent to their offspring [49]. In relation to child health, nutritional epigenetics and behavioural epigenetics are yielding interesting findings. Nutritional epigenetics has started to investigate the effects of breast milk on diseases such as neonatal necrotizing enterocolitis, infectious diseases and the development of obesity [46]. Behavioural epigenetics is a field of epigenetics interested in the study of physiological, genetic, environmental and developmental mechanisms in behaviour investigating the gene expression and processes underlying normal and abnormal behaviour associated with for example, disorders, development and parenting. This area of research is relevant as it provides an opportunity to discuss epigenetic processes that affect normal behaviour [47]. Breastfeeding behaviours such as suckling and skin to skin contact during feeding are thought to be linked to regulating responses to stress and altered epigenetic states. Perhaps one of the exciting features of epigenetics is that these changes may be heritable. Initial findings from research indicate that positive effects resulting from a mother's choice to breastfeed may be passed on to the next generation through our genes [51].

REFERENCES

[1] World Health Organization, United Nations Children's Fund, World Bank Group. *Nurturing care for early childhood development: a framework for helping children survive and thrive to transform health and human potential.* Geneva: World Health Organization, 2018. https://apps.who.int/iris/bitstream/handle/10665/ 272603/9789241514064-eng.pdf.

[2] Britto, Pia Rebello., Patrice L. Engle, and Charles M. Super. 2013. "Early Childhood Development." Translating Research to Global Policy in *Handbook of Early Childhood Development Research and Its Impact on Global Policy.* edited by Pia Rebello Britto, Patrice L. Engle, and Charles M. Super, 3-24. Oxford: Oxford University Press. (Britto, Engle, and Super 2013, 5)

[3] Victora, Cesar G., Rajiv Bahl, Aluísio J. D. Barros, Giovanny V. A. França, Susan Horton, Julia Krasevec, Simon Murch, et al. 2016. "Breastfeeding in the 21st Century: epidemiology, mechanisms, and lifelong effect." *The Lancet* 387:475-490. doi.org/10.1016/S0140-6736(15)01024-7.

[4] Feacham, Richard G., and Marge A. Koblinsky. 1984. "Interventions for the control of diarrhoeal diseases among young children: promotion of breast-feeding." *Bull World Health Organ* 62(2) 271-291. https://www.ncbi.nlm.nih.gov/pmc/articles/PMC2536296/ ?page=1.

[5] World Health Organisation. *"WHO and UNICEF issue new guidance to promote breastfeeding in health facilities globally."*

2018. https://www.who.int/news-room/detail/11-04-2018-who-and-unicef-issue-new-guidance-to-promote-breastfeeding-in-health-facilities-globally.

[6] Dieterich, Christine M., Julia P. Felice, Elizabeth O'Sullivan, and Kathleen M. Rasmussen. 2013. "Breastfeeding and Health Outcomes for the Mother-Infant Dyad." *Pediatr Clin North Am* 60(1):31–48. doi: 10.1016/j.pcl.2012.09.010.

[7] World Health Organisation. *Infant and young child feeding. Model Chapter for textbooks for medical students and allied health professionals.* Geneva: World Health Organisation, 2009. https://apps.who.int/iris/bitstream/handle/10665/44117/9789241597494_eng.pdf?sequence=1&isAllowed=y.

[8] Arenz, S., R. Rückerl, B. Koletzko, and R. von Kries. 2004. "Breastfeeding and childhood obesity—a systematic review." *International Journal of Obesity* 28:1247–1256. https://www.nature.com/articles/0802758.

[9] Uvnäs Moberg, Kerstin., and Danielle K. Prime. 2013. "Oxytocin effects in mothers and infants during breastfeeding." *Infant* 9(6):201-206. http://www.infantjournal.co.uk/pdf/inf_054_ers.pdf.

[10] Innis, Sheila M. 2007. "Fatty acids and early human development." *Early Hum Dev* 83(12):761–766. doi: 10.1016/j.earlhumdev.2007.09.004.

[11] Smith, Stephanie L., and Christopher A. Rouse. 2017. "Docosahexaenoic acid and the preterm infant." *Matern Health Neonatol Perinatol* 3:22. doi: 10.1186/s40748-017-0061-1.

[12] Anderson, J. W., B. M. Johnstone, and D. T. Remley. 1999. "Breastfeeding and cognitive development: a meta-analysis." *Am J Clin Nutr* 70(4):525–535. https://www.ncbi.nlm.nih.gov/pmc/articles/PMC2536296/?page=1.

[13] Horta, Bernardo L., Christian Loret de Mola, and Cesar G. Victora. 2015. "Breastfeeding and intelligence: a systematic review and meta-analysis." *Acta Paediatrica* 104:14-19. https://doi.org/10.1111/apa.13139.

[14] Kramer, Michael S., Frances Aboud, Elena Mironova, Irina Vanilovich, Robert W. Platt, Lidia Matush, et al. 2008. "Breastfeeding and child cognitive development: new evidence from a large randomized trial." *Arch Gen Psychiatry* 65(5):578-84. doi:10.1001/archpsyc.65.5.578.

[15] Goodman, R. 1997. "The Strengths and Difficulties Questionnaire: a research note." *J Child Psychol Psychiatry* 38(5):581–586. doi.org/10.1111/j.1469-7610.1997.tb01545.x.

[16] Girard, Lisa-Christine., Orla Doyle, and Richard E. Tremblay. 2017. "Breastfeeding, Cognitive and Noncognitive Development in Early Childhood: A Population Study." *Pediatrics* 139(4).e2161848 https://pediatrics.aappublications.org/content/139/4/e20161848.

[17] Sullivan, Jerome L. 2008. "Cognitive development: breast-milk benefit vs infant formula hazard." *Arch Gen Psychiatry* 65(12):1456. doi: 10.1001/archpsyc.65.12.1456-a.

[18] Der, Geoff., G. David Batty, and Ian J. Deary, 2006 "Effect of breast feeding on intelligence in children: prospective study, sibling pairs analysis, and meta-analysis." *BMJ* 333:945. doi: https://doi.org/10.1136/bmj.38978.699583.55.

[19] Jacobson, S. W., R. C. Carter, and J. L. Jacobson. 2014. "Breastfeeding as a proxy for benefits of parenting skills for later reading readiness and cognitive competence." *J Pediatr* 164:440–2. doi: 10.1016/j.jpeds.2013.11.041.

[20] Leventakou, Vasiliki., Theano Roumeliotak, Katerina Koutra, Maria Vassilaki, Evangelia Mantzouranis, Panos Bitsios, Manolis, Kogevinas, and Leda Chatzi. 2013. "Breastfeeding duration and cognitive, language and motor development at 18 months of age: Rhea mother–child cohort in Crete, Greece." *Journal of Epidemiology and Community Health* 69(3):232-239. doi.org/10.1136/jech-2013-202500.

[21] Michels, Kara A., Akhgar Ghassabian, Sunni L. Mumford, Rajeshwari Sundaram, Erin M. Bell, Scott C. Bello, and Edwina H. Yeung. 2017. "Breastfeeding and motor development in term and

preterm infants in a longitudinal US cohort." *Am J Clin Nutr* 106:1456–62. doi: 10.3945/ajcn.116.144279.
[22] Dee, Deborah L., Ruowei Li, Li-Ching Lee, and Laurence M. Grummer-Strawn. 2007. "Associations between Breastfeeding Practices and Young Children's Language and Motor Skill Development." *Pediatrics.* 119:592-598 https://pediatrics.aappublications.org/content/119/Supplement_1/S92.
[23] Iqbal, Meesha, Ghazala Rafique, and Sumera Ali. 2017. "The Effect of Breastfeeding on the Cognitive and Language Development of Children Under 3 Years of Age: Results of Balochistan-Early Childhood Development Project." *J Gen Pract* 5:305. doi:10.4172/2329-9126.1000305.
[24] UNICEF. *"Skin to Skin Contact."* 2019. https://www.unicef.org.uk/babyfriendly/baby-friendly-resources/implementing-standards-resources/skin-to-skin-contact/.
[25] Sal, F. S. 2005. "The role of the mother's voice in developing mother's face preference: Evidence for intermodal perception at birth." *Infant Child Development* 14:29-50. https://doi.org/10.1002/icd.376.
[26] UNICEF. "Responsive Feeding Infosheet." 2019. https://www.unicef.org.uk/babyfriendly/baby-friendly-resources/relationship-building-resources/responsive-feeding-infosheet/.
[27] UNICEF. "Responsive Feeding Infosheet: Supporting close and loving relationships." 2019. https://www.unicef.org.uk/babyfriendly/baby-friendly-resources/relationship-building-resources/responsive-feeding- infosheet/.
[28] Tharner, A., M. P. Luijk, H. Raat, M. H. Ijzendoorn, M. J. Bakermans-Kranenburg, H. A. Moll, V. W. Jaddoe, A. Hofman, F. C. Verhulst, and H. Tiemeier. 2012. "Breastfeeding and its relation to maternal sensitivity and infant attachment." *Dev Behav Pediatr* 33:396-404. doi: 10.1097/DBP.0b013e318257fac3.
[29] Tharner, Anne., Maartje P. C. M. Luijk, Hein Raat, Marinus H. IJzendoorn, Marian J. Bakermans-Kranenburg, Henriette A. Moll,

Vincent W. V. Jaddoe, et al. 2012. "Breastfeeding and Its Relation to Maternal Sensitivity and Infant Attachment." *Journal of Developmental & Behavioral Pediatrics* 33(5):396–404. doi:10.1097/DBP.0b013e318257fac3.

[30] Ventura, Alison K. 2017. "Associations between Breastfeeding and Maternal Responsiveness: A Systematic Review of the Literature." *Advances in Nutrition* 8:495–510. doi.org/10.3945/an.116.014753.

[31] Brazelton, T. B., B. Koslowski, and M. Main. 1974. "The origins of reciprocity: The early mother-infant interaction." In *The effect of the infant on its caregiver*. M. Lewis and L. A. Rosenblum. Oxford: Wiley-Interscience.

[32] Douglas, Hazel. 2007. *Containment and Reciprocity: Integrated psychoanalytic theory and child development for work with children.* East Sussex: Routledge.

[33] Brazelton, T., and B. G. Cramer. 1991. *The Earliest Relationship.* London: Karnac.

[34] Tonse, N. K. Raju. 2011. "Breastfeeding Is a Dynamic Biological Process—Not Simply a Meal at the Breast." *Breastfeed Med* 6(5):257–259. doi: 10.1089/bfm.2011.0081.

[35] Douglas, Hazel. 2017. *The First Five Years: Solihull Approach Resource Pack.* Cambridge: Jill Rodgers Associates.

[36] Rheeston, Mary. 2018. "The Solihull Approach and Peer Breastfeeding Supporter training." In *The Solihull Approach in Practice,* edited by Hazel Douglas, 77-85. Solihull: Solihull Approach. (Rheeston 2018, 77)

[37] Anothaisintawee, T., C. Wiratkapun, P. Lerdsitthichai, V. Kasamesup, S. Wongwaisayawan, J. Srinakarin, S. Hirunpat, et al. 2013. "Risk factors of breast cancer: a systematic review and meta-analysis." *Asia Pac J Public Health* 25(5):368-87. doi: 10.1177/1010539513488795.

[38] Zhou, Ying., Jingde Chen, Qun Li, Wei Huang, Haifeng Lan, and Hong Jiang. 2015. "Association Between Breastfeeding and Breast Cancer Risk: Evidence from a Meta-analysis." *Breastfeeding Medicine* 10(3):175-82. doi.org/10.1089/bfm.2014.0141.

[39] World Cancer Research Fund. *"Diet Nutrition, Physical Activity and Breast Cancer."* 2018. http://www.aicr.org/continuous-update-project/reports/breast-cancer-report-2017.pdf.

[40] Modugno, Francesmary., Sharon L. Goughnour, Danielle Wallack, Robert P. Edwards, Kunle Odunsi, Joseph L. Kelley, Kirsten Moysich, Roberta B. Ness, and Maria Mori Brooks. "Breastfeeding factors and risk of epithelial ovarian cancer." 2019 *Gynecologic Oncology* 25:116-22.https://read.qxmd.com/read/30686553/breastfeeding-factors-and-risk-of-epithelial-ovarian-cancer.

[41] Gunderson, Erica P., Cora E. Lewis, Ying Lin, Mike Sorel, Myron Gross, Stephen Sidney, David R. Jacobs Jr, James M. Shikany, and Charles P. Quesenberry Jr. 2018. "Lactation Duration and Progression to Diabetes in Women Across the Childbearing Years." *AMA Intern Med* 178(3):328-337. doi:10.1001/jamainternmed.2017.7978.

[42] Department of Health. *"Early Intervention Transformation Programme."* 2018. https://www.health-ni.gov.uk/articles/early-intervention-transformation-programme.

[43] Rheeston, Mary. 2018. "The Solihull Approach in the Antenatal and Postnatal Period." In *The Solihull Approach in Practice,* edited by Hazel Douglas, 51-58. Solihull: Solihull Approach. (Rheeston 2018, 53-55)

[44] Northern Ireland Assembly. "Breastfeeding: Attitudes and Policy." *Research and Information Briefing Paper.* 25 January 2017. http://www.niassembly.gov.uk/globalassets/documents/raise/publications/2016-2021/2017/health/0917.pdf.

[45] Shakya Prakash., Mika Kondo Kunieda, Momoko Koyama, Sarju Sing Rai, Moe Miyaguchi, Sumi Dhakal, Su Sandy, Bruno Fokas Sunguya, and Masamine Jimba. 2017. "Effectiveness of community-based peer support for mothers to improve their breastfeeding practices: A systematic review and meta-analysis." *PLoS One* 12(5): e0177434. doi: 10.1371/journal.pone.0177434.

[46] Thomson, Gill, Nicola Crossland, and Fiona Dykes. 2012. "Giving me hope: women's reflections on a breastfeeding peer support service." *Maternal and Child Nutrition* 8(3):340-353. doi.org/10.1111/j.1740-8709.2011.00358.x.

[47] Tan, Monique, Mary Rheeston, and Hazel Douglas. 2017. "Using the Solihull Approach in breastfeeding support groups: Maternal perception." *British Journal of Midwifery* 25(12):765-773.

[48] Thelwell, E., Mary Rheeston, and Hazel Douglas. 2017. "Exploring breastfeeding peer supporters' experience of using the Solihull Approach model." *British Journal of Midwifery* 25(10):639-655.

[49] Deans, Carrie, and Keith A. Maggert 2015. "What Do You Mean, "Epigenetic?" *Genetics* 199(4):887–896. doi: 10.1534/genetics.114.173492.

[50] Verduci, Elvira, Giuseppe Banderali, Salvatore Barberi, Giovanni Radaelli, Alessandra Lops, Federica Betti, Enrica Riva, and Marcello Giovannini. 2014. "Epigenetic Effects of Human Breast Milk." *Nutrients* 6(4):1711–1724. doi: 10.3390/nu6041711.

[51] Lester, Barry M., Edward Tronick, Eric Nestler, Ted Abel, Barry Kosofsky, Christopher W. Kuzawa, Carmen J. Marsit, et al. 2011. "Behavioral epigenetics." *Ann N Y Acad Sci* 1226:14–33. doi: 10.1111/j.1749-6632.2011.06037.x.

In: New Research on Breastfeeding ...
Editor: Kai Santos Melo

ISBN: 978-1-53617-061-0
© 2020 Nova Science Publishers, Inc.

Chapter 2

BREAST MILK FOR PREMATURE INFANTS: NUTRITIVE AND HEALTH ASPECTS

Nikoleta M. Lugonja, PhD and Snežana D. Spasić, PhD*
Department of Chemistry,
Institute of Chemistry, Technology and Metallurgy,
University of Belgrade, Belgrade, Serbia

ABSTRACT

Breast milk is considered to be the only and the best nutrition for newborn infants until six months of age. However, some of the most important problems regarding the nutrition of infants after preterm delivery are due to the fact that preterm milk is produced before complete maturation of mammary glands and that the preterm infant's gastrointestinal tract is not mature enough at the time of partition. Since human milk has unique properties in promoting gastrointestinal maturation and immunological benefits, it is very important to implement strategies of fortification to appropriately actuate its benefits. Donor breast milk from milk banks is widely used when mother's own milk is

---

* Corresponding Author's Email: nikoleta@chem.bg.ac.rs.

not available or when it is in short supply for preterm infants. While donor breast milk retains some of the biological properties and clinical benefits of mother's own milk, it requires additional care in terms of fortification, especially if the donor milk is from a pool of term breast milk which is somewhat different than preterm breast milk.

As nutritional strategies improve, the ultimate goal is to minimize extrauterine growth restriction and promote appropriate growth and development of premature infants. Another problem with breast milk, which is quite often overlooked, is that after six months, there is not enough of essential microelements (Zn, Fe and Cu) to satisfy baby's needs, and therefore, the milk must be effectively supplemented.

In this chapter we review the following aspects of breast milk for preterm infants: 1) The main nutritive factors of breast milk; 2) The use of fortifier as breast milk supplement; 3) Significance of microelements in preterm nutrition; and 4) Health outcomes of breast milk for preterm infants.

Keywords: breast milk, infant nutrition, premature infants

INTRODUCTION

The composition of breast milk (BM) is specially adapted to the infant's needs. Based on its nutritional composition and biological activity, breast milk is considered to be the "gold standard" in infant nutrition. The implementation of human breast milk (BM) in the diet of preterm babies is very significant, which is in line with WHO recommendations for the use of breast milk or pasteurized donor milk in the early diet of preterm babies, which begins in neonatal units (WHO, 2011). Nutrition is one of the crucial factors that influence the growth and developmental characteristics of preterm infants. There is also a need to fundamentally provide adequate nutrition in the early days of preterm infant's life with a well-balanced parenteral and enteral nutrition strategy to reduce extra-uterine growth retardation in very-low-birth-weight infants (VLBW). Providing adequate amounts of nutrients helps to improve early growth, as well as long-term neurocognitive development (Mangili et al., 2017).

Premature breast milk (PBM) nutrition has been linked to a number of beneficial effects and it is a key component in the strategy of enteral nutrition for preterm infants (Boquien, 2018; Lönnerdal, 2000). In addition to nutritional factors, BM has biologically important ingredients, immunoglobulins, non-antibody mediated immune factors, digestive enzymes, growth factors and hormones that can influence growth and development, and are regulated by neuroendocrine and immune factors controlled by the biological clock (Gartner, 2005).

Breast milk also affects the development and reduction of frequent complications in preterm infants, such as NEC and bronchopulmonary dysplasia. Numerous beneficial effects of HM nutrition, manifested at a later age, significantly reduce the risk of developing "metabolic syndrome" and have been the subject of numerous research studies (Arslanoglu et al., 2010).

The nutrient requirements of premature infants differ significantly based on the stage of prematurity. The variations in the composition of preterm and term human milks are caused by a variety of reasons including early pregnancy interruption and variable hormonal profiles (Bhatia, 2013). The average nutrient levels in preterm breast milk do not meet the increased nutritional requirements of preterm infants. Feeding premature infants exclusively with HM over a longer period is associated with poorer growth and progression, as well as the development of a nutritional deficit compared to a group fed with enriched BM or an infant formula for premature infants (Lönnerdal, 2000). Using fortifier to supplement breast milk, it is possible to feed premature infants BM, which has many positive effects, and fulfill of the specific nutritional needs of preterm infants in accordance with the recommendations of The European Society for Pediatric Gastroenterology Hepatology and Nutrition (ESPGHAN) (ESPGHAN, 2013).

1. THE MAIN NUTRITIVE FACTORS OF BREAST MILK

Breast milk is very variable and its composition is adapted to the needs of the baby. Breast milk consists of 87% water, 0.8-0.9% protein, 3-5% lipid, 6.9-7.2% carbohydrates and 0.2% minerals and vitamins. Depending on the time of secretion and composition, we distinguish colostrums, transient and mature milk (Jenness 1979; Gidrewicz & Fenton, 2014). Carbohydrates, lipids and proteins are the major components that contribute to the energy content of 60-75 kCal/100 mL in human milk (WHO 2001 & 2002).

There are differences in the composition of milk from women who deliver prematurely and women who deliver at term. Although protein content in colostrum of preterm milk is significantly higher than term milk, it changes and decreases in the weeks after delivery, while fat and lactose content vary over the lactation period, as well as from the start to the end of feeding. Preterm breast milk has initially higher concentrations of protein, fat, free amino acids and sodium and lower lactose concentrations, but these concentrations decline after the first weeks after delivery (Bauer & Gerss, 2011). However, the content of macronutrients may be inadequate due to the difference in the individual composition of breast milk. Low protein content, low sodium, calcium and phosphorus concentrations below the level required for fetal bone mineralization in BM may have an impact on the exclusively BM diet of preterm infants in the long term being associated with poorer growth and progression, as well as the development of nutritional deficits in the ratio to a group fed with an enriched BM or infant formula for premature infants (De Curtis &Rigo, 2012). Proteins and amino acids are essential for the growth and development of infants, especially in preterm infants because of their rapid growth. Preterm infants have greater protein requirements than term infants, and it is important to provide a protein requirement of 3.4–4.3 g/kg/d total protein without distinguishing among the various stages postpartum (Dallas et al., 2012).

1.1. Proteins

The most important breast milk proteins are β-casein and whey proteins, such as α-lactalbumin, lactoferrin, immunoglobulin A (IgA) and serum albumin, each of them consisting of an impressive range of specific proteins and peptides. Preterm mothers' milk has more protein than the milk of mothers who gave birth at term. Protein content changes during lactation. Colostrum and transitional milk have high protein concentrations but with low casein concentration, which increases during the lactation period. Whey protein concentrations remain high throughout the lactation period (Stam et al., 2013). Whey proteins are synthesized in mammary gland, while other proteins such as serum albumin, various enzymes and protein hormones are transferred to milk from plasma. The dimer of secretory IgA is synthesized in mammary gland epithelial cells and then resident lymphocytes connect two IgA molecules (Golinelli et al., 2014). During the first 8 weeks of lactation, the protein content of women who have given birth is higher, and the protein concentration being inversely correlated with gestational age. According to research of Bauer & Gerss average protein concentration of milks from term and premature mothers differs over the first eight weeks of lactation: extremely preterm human milk 2.8 ± 0.5 g/dL (<28 weeks), severely preterm human milk 2.1 ± 0.3 g/dL (28-31 weeks), moderately preterm human milk 1.9 ± 0.3 g/dL (32-33 weeks), and term human milk 1.6 ± 0.5 g/dL. During lactation, the milk protein content decreases in both women delivering prematurely and at term (Bauer & Gerss, 2011). Human milk contains active proteases, protease precursors, inhibitors and activators, which are active in the infant stomach, but they are not instrumental in overall gastric digestion in either preterm or term infants. Preterm infant's overall lower gastric protein digestion cannot be compensated by enzymes in preterm milk (Demers-Mathieu et al., 2018). Decreasing protein content in preterm milk during lactation can cause a decrease in growth in exclusively breastfed infants compared to formula-fed infants. Preterm infants are capable of degrading human milk proteins regardless of prematurity and postnatal age, with limited contribution of milk protease to protein digestion (Gianni et al., 2019).

In preterm infants, human milk provides immunological benefits via two mechanisms: the direct action of lactoferrin, lysozyme, defensin and cytokines, and a high concentration of growth factors and nucleotides that stimulate the immune system (Lewis et al., 2017). In addition to these functions, proteins and peptides in milk also play a role in the antioxidant protection of infants. Several studies have been done to show that the antioxidant activity of proteins and peptides is associated with their amino acid composition (tyrosine, tryptophan, methionine, lysine, cysteine, phenylalanine and hystidine). The mechanisms of antioxidant activity of proteins and peptides are the result of a combination of scavenging of free radicals, inhibition of lipid peroxidation, and chelating of transition metal ions (Pihlanto, 2016).

1.2. Lipids

Lipids are macronutrients that provide 50% of the energy for the infant, essential for the growth and development of the infant's brain (Bernard et al., 2017; Prentice et al., 2016). During the lactation, total fat in breast milk changes and adapts in accordance with the environment, diet and physiological state of the mother. Compared to colostrums with a low content of fat in both preterm or term milk, fat content in the mature milk increased by approximately one half in preterm milk or doubled in term milk (Thakkar et al., 2013; Gidrewicz& Fenton, 2014). Hindmilk, defined as the last milk of a feed, may contain two to three times the concentration of milk fat found in foremilk, defined as the initial milk of a feed (Saarela et al., 2005). Kent et al., examined fat content of breast milk throughout 24-hour period and found that the milk fat content was significantly lower in night and morning feedings compared to afternoon or evening feedings (Kent et al., 2006).

Breast milk contains lipids in the form of triacylglycerol (TAG), with high concentrations of long-chain fatty acids, palmitic and oleic, the former heavily concentrated in the 2-position and the latter in the 1- and 3- positions of the triglycerides. Linoleic acid (LA) and α-linolenic acid (ALA) in BM are precursors of long-chain polyunsaturated fatty acids (PUFAs) ω6 and ω3 (arachidonic acids and eicosapentaenoic and docosahexaenoic acids (DHA)). These precursors are not synthesized in vivo and breast. Breast milk also contains cholesterol, which is a hormone precursor and together with PUFA and DHA, it is essential for brain development (Boquien, 2018). Researches had shown that fatty acids in breast milk can be modified by maternal nutrition or nutritional supplementation, but this does not affect the amount or concentration of total lipids (Innis, 2014).

There are differences in the fat content of preterm and term milk. Preterm milk contains significantly more fat than term milk and shows a further increase during lactation. The high fat content is responsible for the higher energy density of preterm milk, since there are higher contents of long and medium chain fatty acids, and smaller size distribution of fat globules in preterm, inversely related to gestational age at delivery. Breast milk also contains enzymes for fat digestion (Lee et al., 2018).

1.3. Carbohydrates

The carbohydrate fraction of human milk is composed of lactose (90-95%) and oligosaccharides (5-10%). Lactose is the most represented energy-providing macronutrient in breast milk. During lactation, lactose concentration in breast milk changes and depends on various factors associated with mother's body mass index (BMI), duration of lactation, etc. Relatively low lactose concentrations are found in colostrum, but they increase significantly during lactation, especially in mothers of preterm infants. The lactose content of human milk rises from 55 g/L to 70 g/L in mature milk. Premature milk lactose content is significantly lower compared to term milk, in colostrums in the first 3 days and a few times later (Gidrewicz & Fenton, 2014). Maintaining glucose homeostasis is not easy in preterm infants because of the increased risk of hypoglycemia, which occurs due to the immaturity of organs involved in glucose metabolism, but it is at the same time exposed to many risk factors for hyperglycemia (insulin resistance, sepsis, limited glucose oxidation) (Koletzko et al., 2005).

In addition to lactose, breast milk oligosaccharides (HMO) are complex carbohydrates that are produced in large quantities and with different structures in breast milk. HMO are high in breast milk, 10 to 20 g/L and have different biochemical composition and structural diversity, with over 130 different structures. HMO contain terminal Gal-β-1,4–Glc, with 3 to 14 monosaccharide units, and in BM, they are present as free structures or conjugated macromolecules, in the form of glycoproteins, glycolipids, etc. (Bode, 2006). HMO are non-nutritive bioactive factors with three important functions: the prebiotic effect when HMO selectively stimulate the growth and activity of bacterial species, competitively bind and inhibit pathogens because they are structurally similar to enterocyte glycans, and provide fucose and sialic acid that are important in host defense, brain gangliosides and neurodevelopment in the protection of premature newborn against necrotizing enterocolitis (NEC). The amount of HMO in preterm milk is varies significantly, which is a consequence of the genetic diversity of mothers, the variability in the content of fucosylated HMO during the lactation period (Coppa et al., 2011; Bode, 2012; De Leoz et al., 2012).

HMOs in human intestines are resistant to enzymatic digestion as they pass through the small intestine, and when undigested, they are substrates for colon fermentation and stimulate the growth of bacteria. Many intestinal bacteria express glycosidases that metabolize these oligosaccharides. HMOs competitively bind to specific receptors on the surface of mucosal cells and act as protection against a large number of pathogenic bacteria and viruses (Schell et al., 2002).

Preterm infants are at very high risk of inflammatory intestinal diseases (i.e., necrotizing enterocolitis). Various clinical factors affect the development of infant's gut microbiome — birth mode, antibiotic administration, environmental care, as well as breast milk. Breast milk oligosaccharides, microbiome and secretory IgA are very important for human metabolism, diversity of gut microbiote and intestinal health (Bäckhed et al., 2005; Gregory et al., 2016; Zanella et al., 2019). HMO diversity increases in preterm milk during lactation and indicates that immature milk is at the beginning of lactation, which also affects the colonization of infant's gut (Boquien, 2018). The presence of 2' fucosyllactose (2' FL) in human milk indicates that the mother is a secretor, while high number of women delivering preterm, non-secretors, had decline in 2'FL concentration, which may affect the lack of a proactive effect for necrotizing enterocolitis (De Leoz et al., 2012; Underwood et al., 2015).

Breast milk contains an array of mother-specific probiotic and commensal bacteria (the milk microbiota), that selectively use complex and individual oligosaccharides as prebiotics for growth when they reach infant gut. Pasteurization completely eradicates BM bacteria, including lactic acid bacteria and bifidobacteria, potentially displacing or altering the impact of BM microbiota on infant gut colonization. Breast milk *Lactobacillus* and *Bifidobacterium* have different roles in the mother-infant relationship and affect the prevention of pathogen colonization, stimulation of reactive antibody production and establishment of a healthy intestinal microbiome, capable of preventing diabetes, autoimmune disorders, allergies, obesity (Zanella et al., 2019; Fernández et al., 2018).

1.4. Bioactive Components in Breast Milk

Bioactive molecules in breast milk are important for the innate immune system. The largest differences are between preterm and term infant colostrum in cytokine concentration, growth factor and lactoferrin. Breast milk minerals have different biological functions, form essential parts of many enzymes and are important for different molecules and structures. The most important mineral constituents of breast milk are Na, K, Ca, Mg, P and Cl (Jenness, 1979).

The mineral content of preterm milk is similar to that of term milk, but calcium concentrations are significantly lower in preterm milk than term milk and do not increase during lactation. The contents of trace elements Cu and Zn are high in preterm milk but decrease during the lactation period. Infant adsorbs 50% of iron from breast milk is partly because breast milk provides factors that aid absorption (de Figueiredo et al., 2010; Djurovic et al., 2017). In addition to minerals, breast milk contains adequate concentrations of vitamins necessary for normal growth and development, except for vitamins D and K. Vitamin D depots are depleted within 8 weeks after birth, so it is recommended to start vitamin D supplementation in infants who exclusively breastfeed, while higher doses (2000 IU) of supplementation for mothers can meet the needs for 25-OH-D in infants. Vitamin K is essential for the protein involved in blood coagulation. Very low concentrations of vitamin K pass through the placenta to the fetus, so infants have extremely low concentrations and supplementation is recommended (Martin et al., 2016).

2. The Use of Fortifier as Breast Milk Supplement

Preterm infants are born in the third trimester of gestation and miss the placental transfer of nutrients that would create stores for use in the postnatal period, so they have higher nutritional requirements per kg compare to term infants. Breastfeeding for preterm infants is a big challenge, so mothers are encouraged to start frequent pumping for several hours after delivery and 8-12 times per day, providing premature infant milk while in NICU units (Underwood, 2013). Contemporary tendencies indicate the need for the formation of milk banks, which are nutritional support in the diet of premature babies. Although milk collection and storage have been a long-established practice, fortification of breast milk marks a new era in preterm infant's nutrition. Fortifiers (FF) can be quite beneficial for breast milk, because, among other things, they can specifically satisfy the increased nutritional needs of premature infants. Milk bank collect, pasteurize and store breast milk, but the processing of breast milk may change alter its nutritional and redox properties (Bertino et al., 2013).

The composition of human milk varies between individuals and mothers during the lactation period, even in individuals during the day. Multidimensional variation in breast milk composition is maternal adaptation to infant needs, geographic region, and diet (Meredith-Dennis et al., 2018) and affects the protein content and energy. Although breast milk is the recommended standard for all infants, including premature infants, due to its variable composition, it is difficult to assess whether nutrient intake is adequate. Energy-rich nutrients in breast milk can be influenced by various factors related to breast BMI, lactation length, stress (Gidrewicz & Fenton, 2014).

Premature infants are less tolerant of high fluid milk volumes than term infants, and therefore, fortification of preterm breast milk is recommended. In support of breastfeeding, fortifiers for human milk supplementation have been introduced into the diet of preterm infants. Fortification has been developed to supplement key nutrients, especially proteins, calcium, phosphorus and vitamin D, in order to adapt breast milk to the high nutritional needs of this fast-growing infant, which improves growth in length, weight, and head circumference (Agostoni et al, 2010; Kuschel& Harding, 2004). The use of FF enables the preterm infants to be fed with BM with its many positive effects and to preserve the emotional bond between mother and infant, while fulfilling the specific nutritional needs of preterm infants in accordance with the recommendations of ESPGHAN (Arslanoglu et al., 2019). Supplementation of breast milk with fortifier allows mothers to contribute optimal nutrition, enable the advancement of their own infant and manage to maintain lactation, which in most cases would be interrupted.

Recommendation of the World Health Organization (WHO, 2011) the American Academy of Pediatrics (American Academy of Pediatrics, 2012) and the European Society of Pediatric Gastroenterology, Hepatology, and Nutrition (ESPGHAN, 2013) is that mother's own milk is the first choice for nutrition of the preterm infants. When mother's milk is not available or preterm mothers cannot provide an adequate supply, pasteurized donor human milk from an established milk bank should be a good alternative for preterm feeding. Since most of the donor milk comes from term mothers and the milk banks have rigorous standards for screening and testing of potential donors, there are various nutritional, safety, supply and immune protection challenges in providing donor human milk to all premature infants. Donor term milk differs from preterm milk in the first weeks after delivery, having lower content of protein, fat and bioactive molecules (Weaver et al., 2019). Holder pasteurization of milk, as a standard in procedure to minimize the potential transfer of infectious agents adversely affects the bioactive components of human milk, enzymatic and non-enzymatic antioxidant systems in breast milk, and also influences a decrease in protein concentration due to loss of IgA, IgM, lactoferrin. The effects of pasteurization and freezing cause a variety of physico-chemical processes leading to changes in breast milk components and affect antioxidant components which can be compensated by the addition of fortifier (Marinkovic et al., 2015).

The European Milk Bank Association (EMBA) working group offered approaches, definitions, suggestions and recommendations for fortification of breast milk. Standard Fortification method is the most utilized regiment in neonatal intensive care units and it implies addition of a fixed amount of multicomponent fortifier per 100 breast milk in order to achieve the recommended nutrient intakes, including a human milk protein content of 1.5 g/L per 50-100 ml/kg volume of the fed milk. This method provides recommended energy, but it still does not fulfill required protein intakes, given the individual physiological differences in milk and the variability of infant's requirements, and may be insufficient for the very-low-birth-weight infant (Arslanoglu et al., 2019; Arslanoglu et al., 2009).

Individualized methods of fortification have shown to improve protein intakes and growth of infant. Targeted fortification is based on analyze of macronutrient composition of breast milk by milk analyzer and addition of fortifier on real macronutrient composition, effective in some trials, and it needs to be improved. Adjustable fortification is used to modulate the dose of the fortifier based on blood urea nitrogen value, which is a marker of protein nutrition level. This method improves protein intakes and growth and should be considered as a method for optimization of fortification (Mangili, 2017; Radmacher&Adamkin, 2017).

2.1. Total Antioxidant Capacity of Breast Milk for Premature Infants

A very important factor in determining the quality of milk used in the diet of premature babies is the presence of antioxidants (Marinkovic et al.,

2015). Premature babies are exposed to oxidative stress after birth and it is believed that supplementation with enzymatic and non-enzymatic antioxidants can prevent the development of a disease, affect the immune system of the newborn and increase neonatal vitality (Su, 2014). Antioxidant protection mechanisms operate in synergy in most systems, although one may dominate depending on the antioxidant structure and properties. Beside enzymatic systems, many small molecules participate in the prevention of oxidative stress, such as carotene, lipoic acid, enzymatic inhibitors (cyclooxygenases), antioxidant enzymatic cofactors (Se, Coenzyme Q10), ROS/RNS scavengers (Vitamin E and C), and transition metal chelators (Hanson et al., 2016; Ozsurekci&Aykac, 2016).

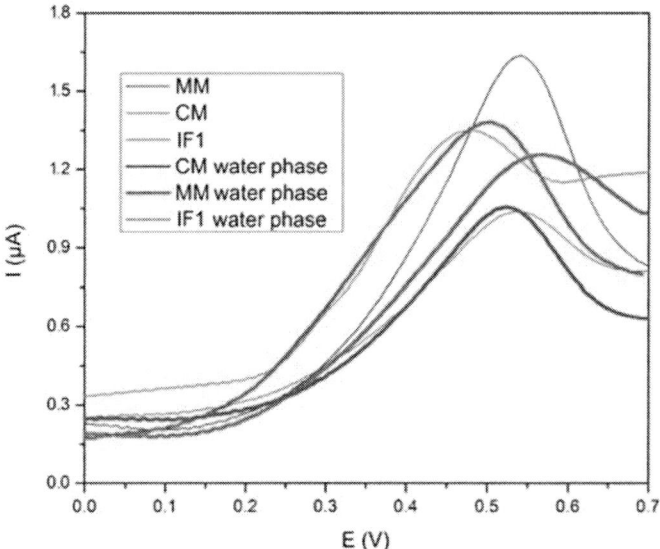

Figure 1. DP voltammograms of milk samples A) Human breast milk–total and water phase (MM), B) infant formula–total and water phase (IF 1), C) commercial UHT milk–total and water phase (CM). The scan rate of 100 mVs−1, pulse amplitude 100 mV, initial potential −400 mV and final potential +1,000 mV (Source: Lugonja et al., (2014) Comparative Electrochemical Determination of Total Antioxidant Activity in Infant Formula with Breast Milk, Food Analytical Methods, 7: 337-344).

Total antioxidant capacity (TAC) can be detected by different methods, and by comparing the measured antioxidant potentials, an overall picture of the action of the antioxidant system, which encompasses the activity of enzymatic and non-enzymatic antioxidants, is obtained. The presence of antioxidants is an essential factor in determining the quality of milk used in the diet of premature infants (Matos et al., 2015).

Breast milk provides better antioxidant protection than infant formulas. Figure 1 shows a comparative study of the total antioxidant potential of human milk, infant formulas and cow's milk (Lugonja et al., 2014). DPV voltammograms show two major reduction peaks that result from redox active reducing species found in the aqueous and fat phase of milk. Higher antioxidant capacity of breast milk is associated with direct scavenging radicals, indicating that breast milk contains more powerful antioxidant system than infant formulas. This is very important for immature defense systems in infants, which become more susceptible to various environmental stressors and in-system fluctuations that are accompanied by increased production of reactive oxygen species. The antioxidant systems that dominate breast milk are vitamins, Fe ions, lactoferrin, as well as the antioxidant activity of specific enzymes superoxide dismutase and glutathione peroxidase. Infant formula development strategy should be based on lowering concentrations of improperly chelated iron and mimicking the composition of small antioxidants molecules of breast milk in order to achieve a more similar composition to breast milk and the dominant role of non-enzymatic components, vitamins A, C, E (Lugonja et al., 2013).

Total antioxidant capacity (TAC) of breast milk can be detected by different methods, and by comparing the measured antioxidant potentials, an overall picture of the action of the antioxidant system is obtained, which encompasses the activity of enzymatic and non-enzymatic antioxidants. A study examining the quality and antioxidant potential of preterm breast milk in the various stages of lactation, storage and pasteurization treatment (Figure 2), indicates that during the process of storage and pasteurization in milk banks, properties and therefore, the quality of milk change (Lugonja et al., 2018).

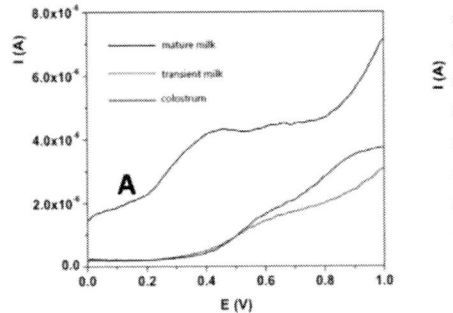 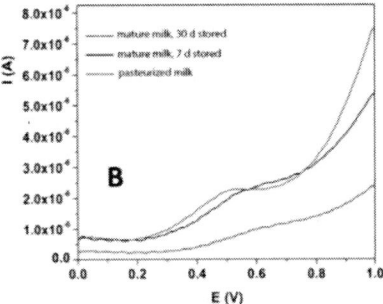

Figure 2. DPV voltammograms: A) Different phases of lactation; and B) Different storage treatment (Source: Lugonja et al., (2018) Electrochemical monitoring of the breast milk quality. *Food Chemistry*, 240: 567-572).

Clinical study of monitoring the breast milk quality showed that colostrums contain higher amounts of reducing agents than transition and mature milks, and that TAC levels decline during lactation period. Investigation of antioxidant potential of breast milk in different lactation phases and after different storage conditions showed that DPV voltammograms were obtained from milks in different lactation phases, and for mature preterm milk, after different storage treatments (Figure 2). The determination of TAC by voltammetric methods can be illustrated by the intensity of the oxidation peak current, which is proportional to the total concentration of the antioxidant compounds. When the DPV was used to examine the milks, one or two oxidation peaks were visible in milk. Areas below reduction peaks are proportional to the quantity of antioxidant compounds in the breast milks. The first peak occurred at around 400 mV, and the second was at 600-700 mV. Colostrum, the product of the first lactation phase, produced oxidation peaks at very high potential, around 800 mV, while mature phase milks produced peak at 500-600 mV. Breast milk with fortifier increased oxidation peak height, proportionally to the antioxidant capacity of milk. However, only one peak was observed at 650-700 mV, similar to the colostrums where peaks at similarly high potentials were also observed. Among the breast milks examined, colostrums contained the greatest level of antioxidant activity. This activity is known to decrease during maturation from colostrum to mature milk, or due to different treatments, causing breast milk to lose scavenging free radicals throughout maturation. Colostrum and mature milk contain different antioxidative systems (Lugonja et al., 2018).

The total antioxidant capacity of preterm milk changes during the lactation period. Exposure of human milk to thermal treatments (pasteurization, freezing) greatly affects the antioxidant status of human milk. Mother's own milk has clear advantages for donor human milk due to its composition and lack of necessity for pasteurization (Marinkovic et al., 2015).

3. SIGNIFICANCE OF MICROELEMENTS IN PRETERM NUTRITION

Nutritional information about human milk is essential as early human growth and development have been closely linked to the status and requirements of several macro- and micro-elements. Recent advances in the neurochemistry of biometals are increasingly establishing the roles of the trace elements iron, copper, zinc, and selenium in a variety of cell functions and are providing insight into the repercussions of deficiencies and excesses of these elements on the development of the central nervous system, especially the limbic system (Tores-Vega et al., 2012).

3.1. Determination of Microelements in Human Milk

Methods addressing the entire mineral profiling in human milk have been scarce due in part to their technical complexities to accurately and simultaneously measure the concentration of micro- and macro-trace elements in low volume of human milk. A single laboratory validation has been performed using a "dilute and shoot" approach for the quantification of sodium (Na), magnesium (Mg), phosphorus (P), potassium (K), calcium (Ca), manganese (Mn), iron (Fe), copper (Cu), zinc (Zn), selenium (Se), molybdenum (Mo) and iodine (I), in both human milk and milk preparations (Dubascoux S et al., 2018). This robust method using new technology ICP-MS/MS without high pressure digestion is adapted to both routinely and rapidly analyse human milk micro-sample (i.e., less than 250 µL) in the frame of clinical trials, but it is also to be extended to the mineral profiling of milk preparations like infant formula and adult nutritionals. In recent data (Pexoto et al., 2019) concentrations of trace elements (Ba, Cu, Fe, Mn, Mo, Se, Sr, and Zn) were determined in human milk, considering the differences between preterm and term human milk and their processing in human milk bank. Significant differences ($p < 0.05$) were found between preterm and term human milk for Ba, Cu, Mo, Se, and Zn, whereas the processing of the donated milk by Holder pasteurization did not influence the concentration of the studied trace elements. The milk of term infants does not offer the recommended daily intake of Zn and for preterm infants the RDI of Fe and Mn is not achieved. The higher concentrations of Cu, Mo, Se and Zn observed in milk from mothers of preterm infants indicate that the milk to be offered to these high-risk neonates in neonatal intensive care units should contain higher levels of these trace elements. Besides, considering the RDI, the milk of term infants should be fortified with Zn, whereas the milk of preterm infants should be fortified with Fe.

Breast milk concentrations of 32 metals and elements in early lactation (days 14-21) were determined in a random sample of first-time Swedish mothers ($n = 60$) using inductively coupled plasma mass spectrometry (ICPMS) (Björklund et al., 2012). There were small inter-individual concentration variations in the macroelements Ca, K, Mg, P and S, and striking similarities across studies and over time, supporting a tight regulation of these elements in breast milk. Large inter-individual and over time differences were detected for Na concentrations, which may reflect an increase in salt consumption in Swedish women. Large inter-individual differences were also detected for the microelements Co, Cr, Mn and Mo, and the toxic metals As, Cd, Pb, Sb and V. Arsenic and B were positively correlated with fish consumption, indicating influence of maternal intake on breast milk concentrations. Observed differences in breast milk element concentrations across studies and over time could be attributed to the timing of sampling and a general decline over time of lactation (Cu, Fe, Mo, Zn), a possible lack of regulation of certain elements in breast milk (As, B, Co, Mn, Se) and time trends in environmental exposure (Pb), or in some cases, to differences in analytical performance (Cr, Fe).

Our results have shown (Figure 3) that FAAS method was more sensitive for Fe determination in human milk, while ICP-OES was more sensitive for both Zn and Cu detection. The limit of quantification for both Zn and Cu was 5 μg/L and 10 μg/L for Fe and the recovery for Zn, Fe and Cu ranged from 90% to 94%, 97% to 103% and 90% to 102%, respectively. Mean concentrations of Zn, Fe, and Cu in human milk samples were 5.35, 0.47 and 0.83 mg/L, respectively, while these values in infant formula ranged from 3.52–4.75 mg/L, 3.37–4.56 mg/L and 0.28–0.41 mg/L, respectively (Djurovic et al., 2017).

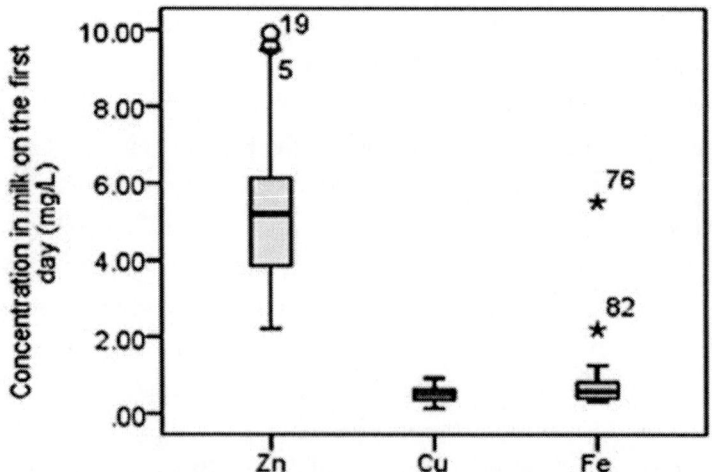

Figure 3. Concentration of Zn, Fe and Cu in human milk samples on the first day after the delivery. The boxes represent the median and the 25th and 75th percentiles; whiskers represent the non-outliner range. (Source: Djurović et al., (2017) Determination of Microelements in Human Milk and Infant Formula without Digestion by ICP-OES, *Acta Chimica Slovenica*, 64(2): 276-282).

There is no statistically significant correlation between Zn, Fe and Cu concentrations in human milk samples. Based on the obtained data and linear regression, it could be concluded that ICP-OES is a better method for Zn determination, FAAS for Fe, while there is no statistically significant difference between these two methods, when Cu is concerned.

Concentrations of microelements in milk are very important for infant nutrition post partum. The results of Se, Zn, and Cu determination in breast milk samples demonstrate a pattern of decline in their concentration with advancing stages of lactation. Wasowicz et al., found that Se, Zn, and Cu concentrations were the highest in colostrum (n = 43) and amounted to 24.8 ± 10.1 µg/L, 8.2 ± 2.8 mg/L, and 0.45 ± 0.11 mg/L, respectively (Wasowiczet al., 2001). The content of all determined microelement declined significantly during the time of lactation. Later, human milk samples were analyzed by neutron activation analysis (NAA) for three essential trace elements Cu, Se, and Zn (Hannan MA et al., 2005). The average concentration level of Cu, Se, and Zn declined from 0.84 ± 0.06 mg/L, 104 ± 9.46 µg/L, and 16.1 ± 2.67 mg/L at day 0 to 0.39 ± 0.045 mg/L, 41.8 ± 6.66 µg/L, and 4.95 ± 1.3 mg/L, respectively, at day 20 of lactation. Cu and Zn levels in the Libyan mothers' milk were in agreement with reported levels from other countries, whereas Se was at a higher level. Se level in the Balkans were reported earlier (Micetić-Turk et al., 2000). Se concentrations were determined by hydride generation atomic absorption spectrometry (HG-AAS). Concentrations of Se in colostrum ranged from 17 to 48 µg/L with a mean of 29 ± 10 µg/L. No significant correlation was found between maternal serum Se concentration and that of colostrum. Analysis of Se concentrations in Greek mothers (68.3 ± 8.5 µg/L) and in their newborns (37.02 ± 8.9 µg/L) were found higher as compared with those in Albanian mothers (37.4 ± 9.9 µg/L) and in their newborns (34.3 ± 9.1 µg/L) ($P < 0.001$). Cu levels were also found higher ($P < 0.001$) in Greek mothers (1687 ± 353 µg/L) and their neonates (449 ± 87 µg/L) compared to those in Albanian mothers (959 ± 318 µg/L) and their newborns (229 ± 67 µg/L). Additionally, 31.5% of neonates born to Albanian women with Se concentrations less than 28 µg/L had higher Se levels ($P < 0.01$) than their mothers (Schulpis KH et al., 2004). The low Se and Cu levels evaluated in the Albanian mothers and their newborns could be related to their poor animal protein intake which could be the consequence of their low socioeconomic status. It is interesting that selenium supplementation of Chinese women with habitually low selenium intake increases plasma selenium, plasma glutathione peroxidase activity and milk selenium, but not milk glutathione peroxidase (GSH-Px) activity (Moore et al., 2000). It was also confirmed that GSH-Px activities in milk did not correlate to the selenium content of the samples (Torres et al., 2003), indicating a crucial role of GSH-Px in control of hydrogen peroxide in human milk. Deficit of Se in Serbia also has no effect on GSH-Px activity in preterm milk.

It has been suggested that the milk of preterm infants should be fortified with Fe. Enteral supplements for premature infants added to human milk to increase nutrient content may induce lipid oxidation due to free radical formation via Fenton chemistry. Iron supplementation may increase oxidative stress in premature infants and they should be given separately from vitamin C-containing supplements (Friel et al., 2007). It is noteworthy that preterm neonates are at increased risk of iron deficiency (Rao et al., 2009).

When copper is concerned, there are also some facts which must be taken into consideration. Copper is a redox-active metal with capacity to form 4–6 coordinate bonds. The concentration of labile copper (various redox-active Cu^{2+} complexes with small ligands) in human milk and other fluids is tightly regulated. However, copper is mobilized in infections, inflammation, and tissue damage (Chaturvedi et al., 2014; Djoko et al., 2015), as well as in a number of other acute conditions, such as neonatal jaundice (Schulpis et al., 2004). Cefaclor reduced Cu^{2+} to Cu^{1+} that further reacted with molecular oxygen to produce hydrogen peroxide. Meropenem underwent degradation in the presence of copper. The analysis of activity against *Escherichia coli* and *Staphylococcus aureus* showed that the effects of meropenem, amoxicillin, ampicillin, and ceftriaxone were significantly hindered in the presence of copper ions. The interactions with copper ions should be taken into account regarding the problem of antibiotic resistance and in the selection of the most efficient antimicrobial therapy for premature infants with altered copper homeostasis (Bozic et al. 2018).

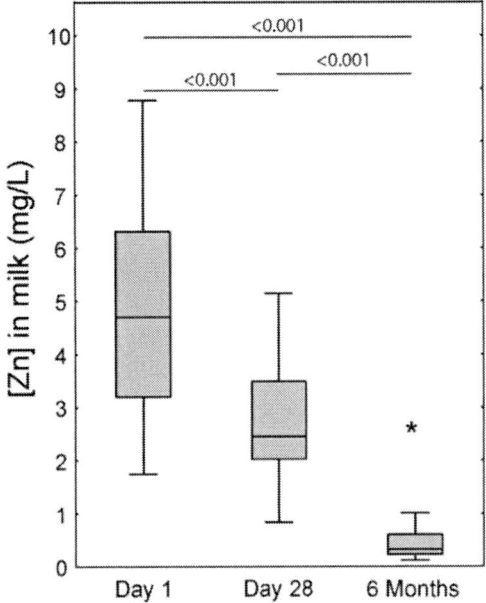

Figure 4. Concentration of Zn in milk during six months after delivery. Boxes represent the median and the 25th and 75th percentiles; whiskers represent the non-outliner range. Outliers (circles) – data point values that are more than 1.5 X IQR outside the box. Extremes (asterisk) – data point more than 3 X IQR outside the box. Statistical significance (p-values) are presented (p > 0.05). (Source: Djurović et al., (2017) "Zinc concentrations in human milk and infant serum during the first six months of lactation" *Journal of Trace Elements in Medicine and Biology*, 41: 75–78.)

Normal supply of zinc to the newborn via milk is essential for normal development. We analyzed changes in the level of Zn in milk and infant serum in the neonatal period (Day 1 and Day 28 post partum) and at 6 months after delivery, in the cohort of 60 mothers and exclusively breastfed babies. The concentration of Zn in the milk showed a decreasing trend during the follow up: Day 1: 4.70 ± 1.74 mg/L; Day 28: 2.65 ± 1.06 mg/L; 6 months: 0.46 ± 0.36 mg/L. The level of Zn in the milk at 6 months of lactation is not sufficient to meet the recommended values (Figure 4) (Djurovic et al., 2017). This implies that in Serbian population, Zn supplementation might also be needed in the later phase of lactation. The amount of Zn available in the milk meets the nutritive requirements during the neonatal period, but a drastic drop at six months of lactation imply that exclusively breastfed infants might be exposed to risk of Zn deficiency.

In living organisms, zinc is redox-inert and has only one valence state: Zn^{2+}. Its coordination environment in proteins is limited by oxygen, nitrogen, and sulfur donors from the side chains of a few amino acids. In an estimated 10% of all human proteins, zinc has a catalytic or structural function and remains bound during the lifetime of the protein. However, in other proteins, zinc ions bind reversibly with dissociation and association rates commensurating with the requirements in regulation, transport, transfer, sensing, signalling, and storage. It is becoming evident that zinc ion speciation is important in zinc biochemistry and for biological recognition, since a variety of low molecular weight zinc complexes have already been implicated in biological processes, e.g., with ATP, glutathione, citrate, or nicotin amine (Krężel & Maret, 2016).

3.2. Effects of Pasteurization and Storage on Trace Elements in Milk

Pasteurization may also have an effect on trace elements. Milk samples were divided into pre- and post-pasteurization aliquots and were Holder pasteurized (Mohd-Taufek N et al., 2016). Inductively coupled plasma mass spectrometry was used to analyze the trace elements zinc (Zn), copper (Cu), selenium (Se), manganese (Mn), iodine (I), iron (Fe), molybdenum (Mo) and bromine (Br). Differences in trace elements pre- and post-pasteurization were analyzed. No significant differences were found between the trace elements tested pre- and post-pasteurization, except for Fe ($P < 0.05$).

It appears that pasteurization- and storage-related loss in the antioxidative activity of ascorbate (Asc) is compensated by uric acid (UA). This is confirmed by increased level of UA radical that is paralleled by decrease in Asc level in the processed milk exposed to oxidation. We found a strong negative correlation (Pearson correlation coefficient r¼0.780, P¼0.002) between UA radical and Asc in raw milk. It has been shown that antioxidative activities of ascorbate and UA are coupled in bovine milk. Ascorbate reacts with UA radical to give rise to UA and Asc (Domazou et al., 2012). This implies that the level of UA radical increases with pasteurization and storage of raw milk, at least partially because of the loss of ascorbate, which is the next in line electron donor.

UA represents a powerful HO· scavenger and repairer of oxidized proteins, whereas UA radical has been shown to scavenge superoxide (Santus et al., 2001). Specific physiological functions of ascorbate, however, cannot be replaced by UA. For example, ascorbate reduces Fe^{3+} to Fe^{2+} to enhance iron absorption in the gut (Lane et al., 2013). UA has the reducing potential of 260 mV and therefore, it can not reduce Fe^{3+} (110 mV at pH 7) (Wardman et al., 1989).

Pasteurization and storage affect nonenzymatic and enzymatic antioxidative agents in human milk (Figure 5). It appears that nonenzymatic antioxidative systems in colostrum and milk are different. The effects of processing may be partially compensated by fortification/spiking with ascorbate before use. Pasteurization had minimal effect on several trace elements in donor breast milk but high levels of inter-donor variability of trace elements were observed. The observed decrease in the iron content of pasteurized donor milk is, however, unlikely to be clinically relevant.

Pregnant and lactating women and infants are vulnerable population groups for adverse effects of toxic metals due to their high nutritional needs and the resultant increased gastrointestinal absorption of both essential and toxic elements. As for the essential element status, only Se levels in maternal serum decreased by 10% in persons who continued smoking during pregnancy compared to non-smokers. In conclusion, the levels of main toxic metals Cd, Pb and Hg and essential elements Ca, Fe, Cu, Zn and Se in maternal blood and three types of breast milk samples in the studied area of coastal Croatia, showed no risk of disrupted essential element levels with regard of toxic metal exposure in both breastfeeding women and their infants (Grzunov-Letinic et al., 2016).

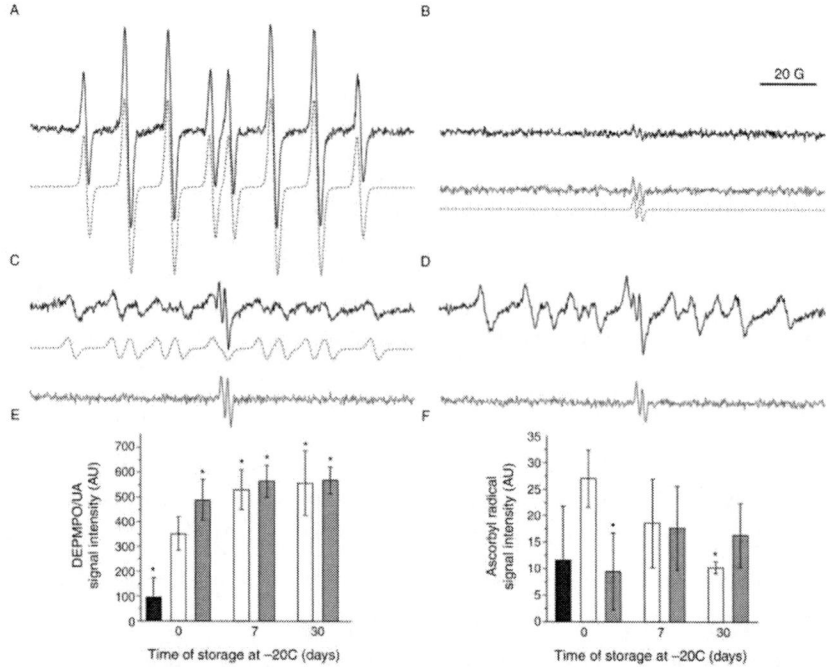

Figure 5. EPR spectra and quantification of redox activity of colostrum and milk exposed to hydroxyl radical-generating system. A, Control system—Fenton reaction: Fe^{2+} (0.6 mM) + H_2O_2 (3 mM). Dotted line—simulation of EPR signal of DEPMPO/OH (signal intensity was 2685 ± 384 AU). B, Colostrum exposed to Fenton reaction. No clear signal of DEPMPO adducts could be identified. Gray line—EPR spectrum obtained in the same system in the absence of spin-trap. Dotted line—simulation of EPR signal of Asc•. C, Fresh milk exposed to Fenton reaction. Dotted line - simulation of EPR signal of DEPMPO/UA. D, Pasteurized milk exposed to Fenton reaction. E, The intensity of EPR signals of DEPMPO/UA adduct. F, The intensity of EPR signals of ascorbyl radical. Black bars—colostrum; white bars—untreated milk; gray bars—pasteurized milk. Statistical analysis was performed using 2-tailed Mann-Whitney (colostrum vs milk) or 2-way ANOVA with post hoc Duncan test (all other data). *= significant compared to untreated human milk at 0 day ($P < 0.05$); ANOVA = analysis of variance; Asc•=ascorbyl radical; AU = arbitrary unit; EPR = electron paramagnetic resonance; DEPMPO=5-(diethoxyphosphoryl)-5-methyl-1-pyrroline-N-oxide; UA= urate. (Source: Marinkovic et al., (2016) "Antioxidative Activity of Colostrum and Human Milk: Effects of Pasteurization and Storage." *Journal of Pediatric Gastroenterology and Nutrition,* 62(6): 901-906.)

4. HEALTH OUTCOMES OF BREAST MILK FOR PRETERM INFANTS

Human milk is generally accepted as the best nutritional choice for newborns and it has been shown to support the optimal growth and development of infants. The composition of human milk is the biologic norm for infant nutrition. Deficiencies of nutrients such as trace elements during gestation and early infanthood have strong deleterious effects on the development of the limbic system; these effects may be irreversible, even when adequate supplementation is provided at later developmental stages (Tores-Vega et al., 2012). In the world, approximately 15% of infants are born preterm (prior to 37 weeks gestation). This is a very heterogeneous population with widely diverse nutritional requirements and highly different stages of immune competence. A 2.5 kg neonate born at 34 weeks gestation differs from a 500-gram neonate born at 24 weeks gestation in essentially every physiologic aspect of the gastrointestinal system and the innate and adaptive immune systems. Perhaps the most compelling benefit of human milk feeding is the observed decrease in necrotizing enterocolitis (NEC). The mechanisms by which human milk protects the premature infant against NEC are most likely multifactorial. The mineral content (including trace minerals) of preterm milk is similar to that of term milk, with the following exceptions: calcium is significantly lower in preterm milk than term milk and does not appear to increase over time, while copper and zinc content are both higher in preterm milk than term milk and decrease during the lactation period. Large inter-individual differences were also detected for the microelements Co, Cr, Mn and Mo, and the toxic metals As, Cd, Pb, Sb and V. As and B were positively correlated with fish consumption, indicating influence of maternal intake on breast milk concentrations. Differences in concentrations present across various studies and over time could be attributed to the timing of sampling and a general decline throughout the lactation period (Cu, Fe, Mo, Zn), a possible lack of regulation of certain elements in breast milk (As, B, Co, Mn, Se) and time trends in environmental exposure (Pb), or in some cases to differences in analytical performance (Cr, Fe) (Björklund et al., 2012).

Previous studies have shown that there are large variations in the level of host defence proteins in individual samples of milk from mothers of premature infants, which implies that large individual variations in antioxidative defence composition are also possible. Our results indicate that transitional milk of mothers of preterm infants shows slow individual variations in antioxidative defence composition; therefore, it can be used in human milk banks. Whey may be its safest fraction for long time preservation and addition of fortifiers (Minic et al., 2018). There are other factors which may influence antioxidative defence in milk. In one study, investigation was done regarding the association between iodine and different markers of oxidative stress and obesity-related hormones in human breast milk (Guterrez-Repisco et al., 2014). That work was composed of two cross-sectional studies (in lactating women and in the general population), one prospective and one *in vitro*. In the cross-sectional study in lactating women, the breast milk iodine correlated negatively with superoxide dismutase (SOD), catalase, and glutathione peroxidase (GSH-Px) activities, and with adiponectin levels. An in vitro culture of human adipocytes with 1M potassium iodide (KI, dose similar to the human breast milk iodine concentration) produced a significant decrease in adiponectin, GSH-Px, SOD1, and SOD2 mRNA expression. However, after 2 months of treatment with KI in the prospective study, a positive correlation was found between 24-h urinary iodine and serum adiponectin. These observations lead to the hypothesis that iodine may be a factor directly involved in the regulation of oxidative stress and adiponectin levels in human breast milk. Factors directly involved in the regulation of oxidative stress are antioxidative enzymes such as superoxide dismutase (SOD), catalase (CAT), glutathione peroxidase (GSH-Px) and glutathione reductase (GR) as well as glutathione (GSH). Colostrum showed almost twofold higher GR activity than mature milk. In accordance with this, Ankrah and colleagues have found a significantly higher level of GSH in colostrum than in mature milk. This might contribute to superior antioxidative performance of colostrums. Substantial loss of GSH occurred when breast milk was kept at either -20°C, 4°C or at room temperature for 2 h (Ankrah et al., 2000). Expressed breast milk showed the progressive loss of antioxidant content, which emphasizes the need of awareness and curtailment of the practice of storing and later use of (Xavier et al., 2011).

Information on breast milk synthesis and its potential defense mechanism against As toxicity are scarce. In one study, purine nucleoside phosphorylase (PNP) and antioxidant enzymes activities, as well as glutathione (GSH) and total arsenic (TAs) concentrations, were quantified in breast milk samples. PNP, superoxide dismutase, catalase, glutathione S-transferase (GST), glutathione peroxidase, glutathione reductase activities and GSH concentration were determined spectrophotometrically; TAs concentration was measured by atomic absorption spectrometry. Data suggest an increase in PNP activity (median = 0.034 U mg/L protein) in the presence of TAs (median = 1.16 g/L). To explain the possible association of PNP activity in breast milk with the activity of the antioxidant enzymes, as well as with GSH and TAs concentrations, generalized linear models were built. In the adjusted model, GSH-Px and GR activities showed a statistically significant ($p < 0.01$) association with PNP activity. These results may suggest that PNP activity increases in the presence of TAs as part of the detoxification mechanism in breast milk (Gaxiola-Robles et al., 2015).

Colostrum contains up to five times more human milk oligosaccharides (HMO) than mature milk. It is tempting to speculate that in addition to their prebiotic and immunological functions, HMO might serve as antioxidants. These human milk oligosaccharides (HMOs) are not digestible by host glycosidases and yet, they are produced in large amounts by the mother with highly variable structures. HMOs appear to have three important functions: prebiotic (stimulation of commensal bacteria containing the bacterial glycosidases to deconstruct and consume the HMOs), decoy (structural similarity to the glycans on enterocytes allows HMOs to competitively bind to pathogens), and provision of fucose and sialic acid that appear to be important in host defense and neurodevelopment, respectively. HMO content of preterm milk varies significantly. Differences between mothers are due to genetic diversity;

there is also a significant variability over time in content of fucosylated HMOs in individual mothers delivering preterm. Glycosaminoglycans (GAG) also appear to act as decoys providing binding sites for pathogenic bacteria to prevent adherence to the enterocyte. Premature milk is richer in GAG than term milk (Underwood, 2013). Bioactive molecules in human milk are important components of the innate immune system. In the early infancy, particularly in premature infants, gastrointestinal tract is not fully developed, which results in incomplete or slow protein digestion. In addition, different proteins might show resistance to proteolysis. For example, it has been found that GSH-Px is not degraded by trypsin or chymotrypsin (protein degradation in small intestine), but it is prone to pepsin (stomach degradation). Hence, at least some amounts of active antioxidative enzymes from the milk might reach infant's intestines. Other physiological functions of these enzymes in intestine, such as the relaxing effects of SOD on smooth musculature, have been proposed (Lugonja et al., 2013). Pertinent to this, SOD and GSH-related enzymes from the milk might be involved in the formation of healthy redox conditions in gut and in the early development of microbiota profile which is known to be sensitive to redox settings.

Amino acid profile is a key aspect of human milk (HM) protein quality. A systematic review of total amino acid (TAA) and free amino acid (FAA) profiles, in term and preterm HM derived from 13 and 19 countries, respectively, was done in a report by Zang et al. (Zang et al., 2013). Effects of gestational age, lactation stage, and geographical region were analyzed by Analysis of Variance. Data on total nitrogen (TN) and TAA composition revealed general inter-study consistency, whereas FAA concentrations varied among studies. TN and all TAA declined in the first two months of lactation and then remained relatively unchanged. In contrast, the FAA glutamic acid and glutamine increased, peaked around three to six months, and then declined. Some significant differences were observed for TAA and FAA, based on gestational age and region. That systematic review represents a useful evaluation of the amino acid composition of human milk, which is valuable for the assessment of protein quality of breast milk substitutes.

The gut ecophysiology in early life may have consequences for the metabolic, immunologic, and even neurologic development of the child, because reports increasingly substantiate the important function of gut microbes in human health. On the basis of scientific insights from human-milk research, a specific mixture of non-digestible oligosaccharides has been developed, with the aim to improve the intestinal microbiota in early life (Oozer et al., 2013). The mixture has been extensively studied and has been shown to be safe and to have potential health benefits that are similar to those of human milk. The specific mixture of short-chain galacto-oligosaccharides and long-chain fructo-oligosaccharides has been found to affect the development of early microbiota and to increase the *Bifidobacterium* amounts as observed in human-milk–fed infants. The resulting gut ecophysiology is characterized by a high concentration of lactate, a slightly acidic pH, and specific short-chain fatty acid profiles, which are high in acetate and low in butyrate and propionate. Lactose is the major carbohydrate in human milk. This disaccharide is an important energy source; it is relatively low in colostrum and increases over time, with more dramatic increases being observed in preterm milk. Complex oligosaccharides are the second most abundant carbohydrate in human milk (Ballard, 2013).

Differences in cytokines, growth factors and lactoferrin between preterm and term milk are the most dramatic in colostrum and early milk and they mostly resolve by 4 weeks after delivery. Leptin is produced by mammary glands, secreted into human milk, and may be important in postnatal growth. Human milk leptin does not appear to differ between preterm and term milk. Bile salt-stimulated lipase activity is similar in term and preterm milk, while lipoprotein lipase activity is higher in term milk. Premature infants that receive human milk have lower rates of metabolic syndrome, lower blood pressure and low-density lipoprotein levels, and less insulin and leptin resistance when they reach adolescence, compared to premature infants receiving formula (Underwood, 2015).

Other potential benefits of human milk to premature infants have been studied with mixed results. The provision of human colostrum in the form of oral care for intubated premature infants has been proposed as a method of stimulating the oropharyngeal-associated lymphatic tissue and altering the oral microbiota, but data to support this intervention are lacking.

Studies of the benefits of human milk in premature infants to date have predominantly compared mother's own milk to premature infant formula. It is unclear whether pasteurized donor human milk (which is generally provided by women who delivered at term) provides similar or superior protection. In premature infants receiving only mother's own milk or pasteurized donor human milk (no formula), increasing amounts of mother's own milk correlate with better weight gain and less NEC. Mother's own milk has clear advantages over donor human milk, both due to its composition and the lack of necessity for pasteurization. Increased efforts to establish and maintain milk supply in women delivering preterm are likely to have greater benefits than providing pasteurized donor human milk. Improved pasteurization protocols and carefully performed trials of galactogogues may be of particular value to this highly vulnerable population (Ballard et al., 2013). Microbial colonization is thought to play an important role in the risk of NEC. Breast feeding is one of many factors that influence the composition of the intestinal microbiota in term infants; limited studies suggest that diet may have less of an effect on the composition of the intestinal microbiota in the premature infant than other factors (such as antibiotic administration). Bioinformatic tools for correlation of the extensive array of fecal metabolites and the fecal microbiota offer great promise in understanding the factors that influence the microbiota of the premature infant (Underwood, 2013). Studies to date suggest that the metabolites differing between human milk-fed and formula-fed infants that are most closely associated with shaping the microbiota include sugars and fatty acids. Whether and how these metabolites differ functionally in the extremely premature infants is unknown.

CONCLUSION

Human milk composition provides the standard for human infant nutrition including the bioactive components that safeguard infant growth and development. Human milk also contains numerous protective bioactive molecules, e.g., lactoferrin, which is being investigated as novel therapeutic agents. These molecules contribute to immune maturation, organ development and healthy microbial colonization of infants.

ACKNOWLEDGMENTS

This work was supported by the Ministry of Education, Science and Technological Development of Republic of Serbia (Project No. III43004).

REFERENCES

Agostoni, C., Buonocore, G., Carnielli, V. P., De Curtis, M., Darmaun, D., Decsi, T., et al., ESPGHAN Committee on Nutrition. (2010). Enteral nutrient supply for preterm infants: commentary from the European Society of Paediatric Gastroenterology, Hepatology and Nutrition Committee on Nutrition. *Journal of Pediatric Gastroenterology and Nutrition,* 50(1): 85-91.

Ankrah, N. A., Appiah-Opong, R., Dzokoto, C. (2000). Human breast milk storage and the glutathione content. *Journal of Tropical Pediatric,* 46(2):111-3.

Arslanoglu, S., Moro, G., Ziegler, E.E. (2009). Preterm infants fed fortified human milk receive less protein than they need. *Journal of Perinatology*, 29: 489-92.

Arslanoglu, S., Bertino, E., Tonetto, P., De Nisi, G., Ambruzzi,A. M., Biasini, A., et al., (2010). Guidelines for the establishment and operation of a donor human milk bank. *The Journal of Maternal – Fetal & Neonatal Medicine*, 23 (2): 1-20.

Arslanoglu, S., Boquien, C. Y., King, C., Lamireau, D., Tonetto, P., Barnett, et al., (2019). Fortification of Human Milk for Preterm Infants: Update and Recommendations of the European Milk Bank Association (EMBA) Working Group on Human Milk Fortification. *Frontiers in Pediatrics*, 7:76.

American Academy of Pediatrics. Section on breastfeeding. (2012). Breastfeeding and the use of human milk. *Pediatrics*, 129: e827–41.

Bäckhed, F., Roswall, J., Peng, Y., Feng, Q., Jia, H., Kovatcheva-Datchary, P., et al., (2005). Dynamics and Stabilization of the Human Gut Microbiome during the First Year of Life. *Cell Host & Microbe*, 17: 690-703.

Ballard, O., Morrow, A. L. (2013). Human Milk Composition: Nutrients and Bioactive Factors. *Pediatric Clinics of North America*, 60(1): 49–74.

Bauer, J., Gerss, J. (2011). Longitudinal analysis of macronutrients and minerals in human milk produced by mothers of preterm infants. *Clinical Nutrition*, 30: 215-220.

Bernard, J. Y., Armand, M., Peyre, H., Garcia, C., Forhan, A., De Agostini, M., Charles, M. A., Heude, B. (2017). EDEN Mother-Child Cohort Study Group. Breastfeeding, polyunsaturated fatty acid levels in colostrum and child intelligence quotient at age 5–6 years. *The Journal of Pediatrics*, 183:43–50.

Bertino, E., Giuliani, F., Baricco, M., Di Nicola, P., Peila, C., Vassia, C., et al., (2013). Benefits of donor milk in the feeding of preterm infants. *Early human development*, 89(2): S3-6.

Bhatia, J. (2013). Human Milk and the Premature Infant. *Annals of Nutrition and Metabolism,* 62(3): 8-14.

Bjorklund, K. L, Vahter, M., Palm, B., Grander, M., Lignell, S., Berglund, M. (2012). Metals and trace element concentrations in breast milk of first time healthy mothers: a biological monitoring study. *Environmental Health*, 11:92.

Bode, L. (2006). Recent advances on structure, metabolism and function of human milk oligosaccharides. The *Journal of Nutrition*, 136: 2127.

Bode, L. (2012). Human milk oligosaccharides: every baby needs a sugar mama. *Glycobiology*, 22(9): 1147–1162.

Boquien, C. Y. (2018). Human Milk: An Ideal Food for Nutrition of Preterm Newborn. *Frontiers in Pediatrics*, 6: 295.

Božić, B., Korać, J., Stanković, D. M., Stanić, M., Romanović, M., Bogdanović Pristov, J., Spasić, S., et al., (2018). Coordination and redox interactions of β-lactam antibiotics with Cu^{2+} in physiological settings and the impact on antibacterial activity. *Free Radical Biology& Medicine,* 129: 279–285.

Chaturvedi, K. S., Henderson, J. P. (2014). Pathogenic adaptations to host-derived antibacterial copper. *Frontiers in Cellular and Infection Microbiology*, 4:3.

Coppa, G. V., Gabrielli, O., Zampini, L., Galeazzi, T., Ficcadenti, A., Padella, L., et al., (2011). Oligosaccharides in 4 different milk groups, Bifidobacteria and Ruminococcus obeum. *Journal of Pediatric Gastroenterology and Nutrition*, 53: 80-87.

Dallas, D., Underwood, M., Zivkovic, A., German, B. (2012). Digestion of Protein in Premature and Term Infants. *Journal of Nutritiona Disorders and Therapy*, 2: 3.

De Curtis, M., Rigo, J. (2012). The nutrition of preterm infants. *Early human development*, 88(1): S5-7.

de Figueiredo, C. S., Palhares, D. B., Melnikov, P., Moura, A. J., dos Santos, S.C. (2010). Zink and Copper concentrations in preterm human milk. *Biological Trace Elements Research*, 136: 1-7.

Demers-Mathieu, V., Qu, Y., Underwood, M. A., Borghese, R., Dallas, D. C. (2018). Premature Infants have Lower Gastric Digestion Capacity for Human Milk Proteins than Term Infants. *Journal of Pediatric Gastroenterology and Nutrition*, 66(5): 816–821.

De Leoz, M. L., Gaerlan, S. C., Strum, J. S., Dimapasoc, L. M., Mirmiran, M., Tancredi, D. J., et al., (2012). Lacto-N-tetraose, fucosylation, and secretor status are highly variable in human milk oligosaccharides from women delivering preterm. *Journal of Proteome Research*, 11 (9):4662–4672.

Djoko, K. Y., Ong, C. L., Walker, M. J., McEwan, A. G. (2015). The role of copper and zinctoxicity in innate immune defense against bacterial pathogens. *The Journal of Biological Chemistry*, 290: 18954–18961.

Djurović, D., Milisavljević, B., Mugoša, B., Lugonja, N., Miletić, S., Spasić, S., Vrvić, M. (2017). Zinc concentrations in human milk and infant serum during the first six months of lactation. *Journal of Trace Elements in Medicine and Biology,* 41: 75-78.

Djurović, D., Milisavljević, B., Nedović-Vuković, M., Potkonjak, B., Spasić, S. D., Vrvić, M. M. (2017). Determination of Microelements in Human Milk and Infant Formula without Digestion by ICP-OES. *Acta Chimica Slovenica*, 64(2): 276-282.

Domazou, A. S., Zhu, H., Koppenol, W. H. (2012). Fast repair of protein radicals by urate. *Free Radical Biology and Medicine*, 52:1929–36.

Dubascoux, S., Andrey, D., Vigo, M., Kastenmayer, P., Poitevin, E. (2018). Validation of a dilute and shoot method for quantification of 12 elements by inductively coupled plasma tandem mass spectrometry in human milk and in cow milk preparations. *Journal of Trace Elements in Medicine and Biology*, 49: 19-26.

ESPGHAN Committee on Nutrition, Arslanoglu, S., Corpeleijn, W., Moro, G., Braegger, C., Campoy, C., Colomb, V., et al., (2013). Donor human milk for preterm infants: current evidence and research directions. *Journal of Pediatric Gastroenterology and Nutrition*, 57: 535–42.

Fernández, L., Ruiz, L., Jara, J., Orgaz, B., Rodríguez, J. M. (2018). Strategies for the Preservation, Restoration and Modulation of the Human Milk Microbiota. Implications for Human Milk Banks and Neonatal Intensive Care Units. *Frontiers in Microbiology*, 9: 2676.

Friel, J. K., Diehl-Jones, W. L., Suh, M., Tsopmo, A., Shirwadkar, V. P. (2007). Impact of iron and vitamin C-containing supplements on preterm human milk: *in vitro*. *Free Radical Biology and Medicine*, 42(10):1591-8.

Gartner, L. M., Morton, J., Lawrence, R. A., Naylor, A. J., O'Hare, D., Schanler, R. J., Eidelman, A. I. (2005). Breastfeeding and the use of human milk. *Pediatrics*, 115: 496-506.

Gaxiola-Robles, R., Labrada-Martagón, V., Kurt Bitzer-Quintero, O., Zenteno-Savín, T., Celina Méndez-Rodríguez, L. (2015). Purine nucleoside phosphorylase and the enzymatic antioxidant defense system in breast milk from women with different levels of arsenic exposure. *Nutricion Hospitalaria*, 31:2289-2296.

Gianni, M. L., Roggero, P., Mosca, F. (2019). Human milk protein vs. formula protein and their use in preterm infants. *Current Opinion in Clinical Nutrition & Metabolic Care*, 22(1): 76-81.

Gidrewicz, D. A., Fenton, T. R. (2014). A systematic review and meta-analysis of the nutrient content of preterm and term breast milk. *BMC Pediatrics*, 14: 216.

Golinelli, L., Mere Del Aguila, E., Paschoalin, V., Silva, J., Conte Junior, C. (2014). Functional aspect of colostrum and whey proteins in human milk. *Journal of Human Nutrition & Food Science,* 2: 1035.

Gregory, K. E., Samuel, B. S., Houghteling, P., Shan, G., Ausubel, F. M., Sadreyev, R. I., Walker, W. A. (2016). Influence of maternal breast milk ingestion on acquisition of the intestinal microbiome in preterm infants. *Microbiome,* 4:68.

Grzunov Letinic, J., Matek Saric, M., Plasek, M., Jurasovic, J., Varnai, V. M., Sulimanec Grgec, A., Orct, T. (2016). Use of human milk in the assessment of toxic exposure and essential element status in breastfeeding women and their infants in coastal Croatia. *Journal of Trace Elements in Medicine and Biology*, 38: 117-125.

Gutierrez-Repiso, C., Velasco, I., Garcia-Escobar, E., Garcia-Serrano, S., Rodrıguez-Pacheco, F., Linares, F., et al., (2014). Does Dietary Iodine Regulate Oxidative Stress and Adiponectin Levels in Human Breast Milk? *Antioxidants & Redox Signaling*, 20: 847–853.

Hannan, M. A., Dogadkin, N. N., Ashur, I. A., Markus, W. M. (2005). Copper, selenium, and zinc concentrations in human milk during the first three weeks of lactation. *Biological Trace Element Research,* 107(1):11-20.

Hanson, C., Lyden, E., Furtado, J., Van Ormer, M., Anderson-Berry, A. A. (2016). Comparison of Nutritional Antioxidant Content in Breast Milk, Donor Milk, and Infant Formulas. *Nutrients*, 8(11): 681.

Innis, S. (2014). Impact of maternal diet on human milk composition and neurological development of infants. *The American Journal of Clinical Nutrition*, 99 (3): 734S–741S.

Jenness, R. (1979). The composititon of human milk. *Seminars in Perinatology*, 3: 225-39.

Kent, J. C., Mitoulas, L. R., Cregan, M. D., Ramsay, D. T., Doherty, D. A., Hartmann, P. E. (2006). Volume and frequency of breastfeedings and fat content of breast milk throughout the day. *Pediatrics*, 117(3): e387–395.

Koletzko, B., Goulet, O., Hunt, J., Krohn, K., Shamir, R., for the Parenteral Nutrition Guidelines Working Group. (2005). Guidelines on Paediatric Parenteral Nutrition of the European Society of Paediatric Gastroenterology, Hepatology and Nutrition (ESPGHAN) and the European Society for Clinical Nutrition and Metabolism (ESPEN), Supported by the European Society of Paediatric Research (ESPR). *Journal of Pediatric Gastroenterology and Nutrition*, 41: S1-S4.

Krężel A, Maret W. (2016) The biological inorganic chemistry of zinc ions. *Arch Biochem Biophys*. 611:3–19.

Kuschel, C., Harding, J. (2004). Multicomponent fortified human milk for promoting growth in preterm infants (Cochrane Review). *Cochrane database of systematic reviews*, 1: CD000343. 10.1002/14651858.CD000343.pub2.

Lane, D. J., Richardson, D.R. (2014). The active role of vitamin C in mammalian iron metabolism: much more than just enhanced iron absorption! *Free Radical Biology and Medicine*, 75: 69–83.

Lee, H., Padhi, E., Hasegawa, Y., Larke, J., Parenti, M., Wang, A., et al., (2018). Compositional Dynamics of the Milk Fat Globule and Its Role in Infant Development. *Frontiers in Pediatrics*, 6: 313.

Lewis, E. D., Richard, C., Larsen, B. M., Field, C. J. (2017). The Importance of Human Milk for Immunity in Preterm Infants. *Clinics in Perinatology*, 44(1): 23-47.

Lönnerdal, B. (2000). Breast milk: A truly functional food. *Nutrition*, *16* (7-8): 509-511.

Lugonja, N., Stanković, D., Spasić, S., Roglic, G., Manojlović, D., Vrvic, M. (2014). Comparative Electrochemical Determination of Total Antioxidant Activity in Infant Formula with Breast Milk. *Food Analytical Methods*, 7: 337-344.

Lugonja, N., Spasic, S., Laugier, O., Nikolic-Kokic, A., Spasojevic, I., Orescanin-Dusic, Z., Vrvic, M. (2013). Differences in direct pharmacologic effects and antioxidative properties of mature breast milk and infant formulas. *Nutrition*, 29: 431-5.

Lugonja, N., Stankovic, D., Milicic, B., Spasic, S., Marinkovic, V., Vrvic, M. (2018). Electrochemical monitoring of the breast milk quality. *Food Chem,* 240: 567-572.

Mangili, G., Garzoli, E. (2017). Feeding of preterm infants and fortification of breast milk. *La Pediatria Medica e Chirurgica*, 39: 158.

Marinkovic, V., Rankovic-Janevski, M., Spasic, S., Nikolic-Kokic, A., Lugonja, N., Djurovic, D., et al., (2015). Antioxidative Activity of Colostrum and Human Milk: Effects of Pasteurization and Storage. *Journal of Pediatric Gastroenterology and Nutrition,* 62: 901–906.

Martin, C. R., Ling, P. R., Blackburn, G. L. (2016). Review of Infant Feeding: Key Features of Breast Milk and Infant Formula. *Nutrients*, 11; 8(5):279.

Matos, C., Ribeiro, M., Guerra, A. (2015). Breastfeeding: Antioxidative properties of breast milk. *Journal of Applied Biomedicine*, 13: 169-180.

Meredith-Dennis, L., Xu, G., Goonatilleke, E., Lebrilla, C. B., Underwood, M. A., Smilowitz, J. T. (2018). Composition and Variation of Macronutrients, Immune Proteins, and Human Milk Oligosaccharides in Human Milk from Nonprofit and Commercial Milk Banks. *Journal of Human Lactation*, *34*(1): 120-129.

Micetić-Turk, D., Rossipal, E., Krachler, M., Li, F. (2000). Maternal selenium status in Slovenia and its impact on the selenium concentration of umbilical cord serum and colostrum. *European Journal of Clinical Nutrition,* 54(6):522-4.

Minić, S., Ješić, M., Đurović, D., Miletić, S., Lugonja, N., Marinković, V., Nikolić-Kokić, A., Spasić, S., Vrvić, M. M. (2018). Redox properties of transitional milk from mothers of preterm infants. *Journal of Paediatrics and Child Health*, 54: 160-164.

Mohd-Taufek, N., Cartwright, D., Davies, M., Hewavitharana, A. K., Koorts, P., McConachy, H., et al., (2016). The effect of pasteurization on trace elements in donor breast milk. *Journal of Perinatology*, 36(10): 897-900.

Moore, M.A., Wander, R. C., Xia, Y. M., Du, S. H., Butler, J. A., Whanger, P. D. (2000). Selenium supplementation of Chinese women with habitually low selenium intake increases plasma selenium, plasma glutathione peroxidise activity, and milk selenium, but not milk glutathione peroxidise activity. *The Journal of Nutritional Biochemistry*, 11: 341–7.

Oozeer, R., van Limpt, K., Ludwig, T., Ben Amor, K., Martin, R., Wind, R., et al., (2013). Intestinal microbiology in early life: specific prebiotics can have similar functionalities as human-milk oligosaccharides. *The American Journal of Clinicl Nutrition*, 98:561S-71S.

Ozsurekci, Y., Aykac, K. (2016). Oxidative Stress Related Diseases in Newborns. *Oxidative Medicine and Cellular Longevity*, 2768365.

Peixoto, R. R., Bianchi Codo, C. R., Lacerda Sanches, V., Guiraldelo, T.C., Ferreira da Silva, F., Ribessi, R.L., et al., (2019). Trace mineral composition of human breast milk from Brazilian mothers. *Journal of Trace Elements in Medicine and Biology*, 54: 199-205.

Pihlanto, A. (2006). Antioxidative peptides derived from milk proteins. *International Dairy Journal*, 16: 1306-1314.

Prentice, P., Ong, K. K., Schoemaker, M. H., van Tol, E. A., Vervoort, J., Hughes, I.A., et al., (2016). Breast milk nutrient content and infancy growth. *Acta Paediatrica*. 105: 641–7.

Radmacher, P. G., Adamkin, D. H. (2017). Fortification of human milk for preterm infants. *Seminars in Fetal and Neonatal Medicine*, 22: 30-5.

Rao, R., Georgieff, M. K. (2009). Iron therapy for preterm infants. *Clinics in Perinatology,* 36:27–42.

Saarela, T., Kokkonen, J., Koivisto, M. (2005). Macronutrient and energy contents of human milk fractions during the first six months of lactation. *Acta Paediatrica,* 94(9):1176–1181.

Santus, R., Patterson, L. K., Filipe, P., Morliere, P., Hug, G. L., Fernandes, A., Maziere, J. C. (2001). Redox reactions of the urate radical/urate couple with the superoxide radical anion, the tryptophan neutral radical and selected flavonoids in neutral aqueous solutions. *Free Radical Research,* 35:129–36.

Schell, M., Karmirantzou, M., Snel, B., Vilanova, D., Berger, B., Pessi, G., et al., (2002). The genome sequence of Bifidobacterium longum reflects its adaptation to the human gastrointestinal tract. *Proceedings of the National Academy of Science of the USA,* 99(22): 14422-7.

Schulpis, K. H., Karakonstantakis, T., Gavrili, S., Costalos, C., Roma, E., Papassotiriou, I. (2004). Serum copper is decreased in premature newborns and increased in newborns withhemolytic jaundice. *Clinical Chemistry,* 50: 1253–1256.

Schulpis, K. H., Karakonstantakis, T., Gavrili, S., Chronopoulou, G., Karikas, G. A., Vlachos, G., Papassotiriou, I. (2004). Maternal-neonatal serum selenium and copper levels in Greeks and Albanians. *European Journal of Clinical Nutrition,* 58(9):1314-8.

Stam, J., Sauer, P., Boehm, G. (2013). Can we define an infant's need from the composition of human milk? *Am J Clinl Nutr,* 98 (2): 521S-528S.

Su, B. H. Optimizing Nutrition in Preterm Infants. *Pediatrics & Neonatology,* 55: 5-13.

Thakkar, S. K., Giuffrida, F., Cristina, C. H., De Castro, C. A., Mukherjee, R., Tran, L.A., et al., (2013). Dynamics of human milk nutrient composition of women from Singapore with a special focus on lipids. *American Journal of Human Biology,* 25(6): 770-9.

Torres, A., Farré, R., Lagarda, M. J., Monleón, J. (2003). Determination of glutathione peroxidase in human milk. *Nahrung,* 47: 430–3.

Torres-Vega, A., Pliego-Rivero, B. F., Otero-Ojeda, G. A., Gomez-Olivan, L. M., Vieyra-Reyes, P. (2012). Limbic system pathologies associated with deficiencies and excesses of the trace elements Iron, Zink, Copper, and Selenium. *Nutrition Reviews,* 70(12): 679-92.

Underwood, M. A. (2013). Human milk for the premature infant. *Pediatric Clinics of North America*, 60(1):189–207.

Underwood, M.A., Gaerlan, S., De Leoz, M. L., Dimapasoc, L., Kalanetra, K. M., Lemay, D. G., et al., (2015). Human milk oligosaccharides in premature infants: absorption, excretion, and influence on the intestinal microbiota. *Pediatric Research*, 78(6): 670-7.

Wardman, P. (1989). Reduction potentials of one-electron couples involving free radicals in aqueous solution. *Journal of Physical and Chemical Reference Data*, 18: 1637–755.

Wasowicz, W., Gromadzinska, J., Szram, K., Rydzynski, K., Cieslak, J., Pietrzak, Z. (2001). Selenium, zinc, and copper concentrations in the blood and milk of lactating women. *Biological Trace Element Research,* 79(3): 221-33.

Weaver, G., Bertino, E., Gebauer, C., Grovslien, A., Mileusnic-Milenovic, R., Arslanoglu, S., et al., (2019). Recommendations for the Establishment and Operation of Human Milk Banks in Europe: A Consensus Statement from the European Milk Bank Association (EMBA). *Frontiers in Pediatrics*, 7: 53.

World Health Organization. *Guidelines on optimal feeding of low birth-weight infants in low- and middle- income countries.* (2011.). www.who.int/maternal_child_adolescent/documents/infant_feeding_low_bw/en).

WHO 2001 & 2002, WHA Res 54 2001 (2001). *The optimal duration of exclusive breastfeeding review, background and meeting report, WHO.* www.ennonline.net/ebfmeeting.

Xavier, A. M., Rai, K., Hegde, A. M. (2011). Total antioxidant concentrations of breastmilk--an eye-opener to the negligent. *Journal of Health, Population and Nutrition,* 29(6): 605-11.

Zanella, A., Silveira, R. C., Roesch, L. F. W., Corso, A. L., Dobbler, P. T., Mai, V., Procianoy, R. (2019). Influence of own mother's milk and different proportions of formula on intestinal microbiota of very preterm newborns. *Plos One*, 14(5): e0217296.

Zhang, Z., Adelman, A. S., Rai, D., Boettcher, J., Lŏnnerdal, B. (2013). Amino Acid Profiles in Term and Preterm Human Milk through Lactation: A Systematic Review. *Nutrients*, 5: 4800-4821.

BIOGRAPHICAL SKETCHES

Nikoleta M. Lugonja, PhD

Affiliation: Assistant Research Professor, Institute of Chemistry, Technology and Metallurgy –Department of Chemistry, University of Belgrade, Serbia

Education:
2005. Graduated from the Faculty of Chemistry, University of Belgrade
2011. MSc degree in Biochemistry, Faculty of Chemistry, University of Belgrade
2014. PhD degree in Biochemistry, Faculty of Chemistry, University of Belgrade

Research and Professional Experience:
Dr. Nikoleta M. Lugonja is assistant research professor with years of diverse experience within field of food chemistry, infant nutrition, biochemistry, microbiology, focusing on food supplements, antioxidants, probiotics and prebiotics.

Professional Appointments:
2008. Teaching Assistant, Faculty of Chemistry, University of Belgrade
2011. Research Assistant, Institute of Chemistry, Technology and Metallurgy, University of Belgrade
2015. Assistant Research Professor, Institute of Chemistry, Technology and Metallurgy, University of Belgrade

Snežana D. Spasić, PhD

Affiliation: Full Research Professor, Institute of Chemistry, Technology and Metallurgy – Department of Chemistry, University of Belgrade, Serbia

Education:
1992. Graduated from the Faculty of Chemistry, University of Belgrade
1998. MSc degree in Chemistry, Faculty of Chemistry, University of Belgrade
2006. PhD degree in Biochemistry, Faculty of Chemistry, University of Belgrade

Research and Professional Experience:
Dr. Snežana D. Spasić is a full researcher professor with years of diverse experience within field of biochemistry, microbiology, biotechnology, food chemistry, focusing on food supplements, antioxidants and metabolic processes.

Professional Appointments:
    1995. Junior Researcher, Institute of Chemistry, Technology and Metallurgy
    1998. Research Assistant, Institute of Chemistry, Technology and Metallurgy, University of Belgrade
    2007. Assistant Research Professor, Institute of Chemistry, Technology and Metallurgy, University of Belgrade
    2013. Associate Research Professor, Institute of Chemistry, Technology and Metallurgy, University of Belgrade
    2018. Full Research Professor, Institute of Chemistry, Technology and Metallurgy, University of Belgrade

In: New Research on Breastfeeding …
Editor: Kai Santos Melo
ISBN: 978-1-53617-061-0
© 2020 Nova Science Publishers, Inc.

Chapter 3

BREASTFEEDING, USE OF COMMON SUBSTANCES AND OFFSPRING'S WEIGHT GAIN AND GROWTH DURING INFANCY AND CHILDHOOD

Edmond D. Shenassa[1], Fiona M. Jardine[2] and Anne Lise Brantsæter[3]

[1]Maternal and Child Health Program, Department of Family Science, and Department of Epidemiology and Biostatistics, University of Maryland, College Park, MD, US
Department of Epidemiology and Biostatistics, School of Medicine, University of Maryland, Baltimore, MD, US
Department of Epidemiology, School of Public Health, Brown University, Providence, RI, US
[2]College of Information Studies, University of Maryland, College Park, MD, US
[3]Department of Environmental Exposure and Epidemiology, Norwegian Institute of Public Health, Oslo, Norway

Among the most important benefits of breastfeeding is the optimal weight gain and growth during infancy that is experienced by infants who are exclusively breastfed for the first six months of life. Appropriate weight gain during infancy is among the most important determinants of healthy development [1]. Infancy weight gain, but not necessarily weight gain during early childhood, has been consistently linked with obesity over the lifecourse [2–5]. Approximately 20% of the risk for becoming overweight during childhood and 30% of the risk for obesity during adulthood is attributable to weight gain during infancy [6]. Because obesity can become intransigent during early childhood, [5] obesogenic processes are best disrupted during pregnancy and infancy, a time of plasticity in neural communication between adipocytes in the brain and other organs and a window of time when the parents are most amenable to changing their behaviors [3].

Influences on infancy weight gain act synergistically and the timing of exposure to these other influences is important. Among the most prevalent influences on infancy weight gain are maternal smoking as well as caffeine intake during and after pregnancy. Direct and secondhand exposure to cannabis[1] is another influence that is gaining in prevalence.

Unfortunately, antismoking programs are of limited availability and have high relapse rates. For this and other related reasons, maternal and paternal smoking during and immediately after pregnancy remains highly prevalent globally. Caffeine intake is similarly prevalent due to its social acceptability and ubiquity. Although cannabis use is not yet as widespread as these other substances, its use is increasing due to its rise in popularity and growing legality. While we have a reasonably good understanding of the effects of smoking and caffeine intake during and after pregnancy, our understanding of their interactions with breastfeeding and their timing remains rudimentary at best. Our understanding of effects of cannabis exposure is even more limited, but enough research now exists to draw

---

[1] Academic literature uses both *cannabis* and *marijuana*. Cannabis is used in this chapter for several reasons: cannabis is the scientific name of the plant, refers to a wider range of cannabinoid-containing products, and does not have a history of being used as a xenophobic, racist trope [125].

preliminary conclusions. A better understanding of how these determinants may interact with breastfeeding to influence weight gain and growth during infancy and childhood can inform interventions to promote optimum infant development.

Current knowledge on each substance will be discussed in terms of prevalence and sources of intake, bioavailability, exposure through breastfeeding and how that may influence weight gain and growth during infancy and childhood, and whether the timing of that exposure may alter those outcomes.

NICOTINE

Prevalence and Sources of Intake

In the United States alone, conservative estimates suggest that 8% of pregnant women (330,000 women in 2014) smoke during their pregnancy [7]. Smoking cessation programs for pregnant women and their partners are not readily available [8]. When available, these programs prove ineffective for majority of the participants, the most successful of these programs achieve quit rates of about 35% by *late* pregnancy [9, 10]. Furthermore, FDA-approved pharmacotherapies are generally not recommended for pregnant or breastfeeding women [11–13]. For these and other related reasons, smoking during and immediately after pregnancy remains highly prevalent in the United States and throughout the world [14, 15].

Bioavailability

Tobacco metabolites, such as cotinine, are readily available in breast milk [16, 17]. The urinary excretion of cotinine (the main metabolite of nicotine) by breastfed infants is comparable to that of adult smokers, and about 10-fold higher than among formula-fed infants, providing clear evidence of the bioavailability of tobacco metabolites in breast milk [18]. Infants exposed to tobacco metabolites gain more weight than other infants, [19, 20] with negative health consequences throughout the lifespan [1, 21]. Thus, a potential consequence of exposure to tobacco metabolites via breast milk may be excessive weight gain during infancy. Evidence from animal studies suggests that exposure to tobacco metabolites, particularly nicotine, during the period of maternal milk feeding is associated with higher adiposity and accelerated growth, possibly even after weaning.

A number of pathways exist by which tobacco metabolites may affect infant weight gain and growth. Milk from smokers contains higher levels of certain polyunsaturated fatty acids compared to nonsmokers, [22] and exposure to polyunsaturated fatty acids is associated with higher fat mass and growth during infancy [23]. Other possible pathways include direct influences of nicotine on the infant's hypothalamus function related to appetite control, [24] placental and fetal hormones (e.g., growth hormone, insulin-like growth factor, and leptin), [25] and weight gain associated with nicotine withdrawal, similar to that observed in adults who quit smoking [26].

Nicotine Exposure through Breastfeeding, Weight Gain and Growth during Infancy and Childhood

Only four studies [27–30] have examined infancy weight gain in the context of both feeding method and exposure to cigarette smoke. Among members of a Seattle health maintenance organization (N = 333; 1982–1983), [28] infants who were breastfed by smokers gained weight more rapidly than infants formula fed by smokers or breastfed by nonsmokers. In contrast, among a nationally representative sample of Dutch women and their infants (N = 1,823; 1988-1989), [29] the effect of exposure to cigarette smoke on infancy weight gain did not vary by feeding method. This discrepancy has been attributed to differences between the participants in the two studies [30]. The study conducted in Seattle preferentially recruited women who had a minimum of two alcoholic drinks per day during their pregnancy; and the prevalence of smokers in this sample (41%) was about 5 times higher than that of the Dutch sample (8%). Smokers in the Seattle sample also smoked more heavily than their Dutch counterparts. The much higher prevalence of heavy smokers in the Seattle sample likely resulted in a higher prevalence of small for gestational age (SGA) infants among this group compared with the Dutch sample. Growth restricted infants, such as those born SGA, are more likely than others to gain more weight during infancy [31]. The effect of exposure to cigarette smoke on weight gain is best examined separately among SGA and appropriate for gestational age (AGA) infants, but neither of these two studies conducted stratified analyses in this manner. Among AGA infants (N = 23,571) in a U.S. historic cohort (1959–1965), exposure to cigarette smoke was not associated with differential infancy weight gain by feeding method, but among the SGA infants (N = 2,552) fetal or postnatal exposure to heavy smoking (≥20 cigarettes per day) predicted significant additional weight gain [30]. Finally, among a hospital-based U.S. sample (N = 813; 2010–2014), breastfeeding protected against risk of excessive weight gain associated with exposure to secondhand smoke (SHS) [27].

Of these four studies, only one study estimated the specific effects of postnatal versus prenatal exposure [30]. However, this study utilized proxy measures for both smoking and feeding method. In sum, currently there are no studies that assess the *specific* effects of postnatal and prenatal exposures on infancy weight gain utilizing data that is prospectively collected directly from mothers and infants. Furthermore, estimation of specific effects of pre- and postnatal exposures requires fitting of an interaction term in the regression models; the relatively small samples of existing studies do not allow adequate statistical power to obtain stable estimates from interaction terms. Similarly, estimation of the effect of exposure to lower levels of cigarette smoke also requires a large analytic sample.

Timing of Exposure

With regard to timing of exposure, practically all of the women who smoke during pregnancy continue to do so after pregnancy; [32] thus, exposing their offspring to SHS during infancy. Evidence suggests that infants exposed to SHS gain more weight than other infants [32]. Differences in physiologic processes that distinguish fetal development from later development suggest the possibility of distinct effects of maternal smoking depending on the time of exposure (i.e., during versus after pregnancy). This hypothesis is further supported by evidence that in utero exposure to maternal smoking and postnatal exposure to SHS each have independent negative effect on other outcomes, such as pulmonary function [33]. Existence of distinct and time-dependent influences is also consistent with evidence from experimental studies. Laboratory animals exhibit distinct physiologic responses to tobacco smoke depending on whether they are exposed during fetal or infantile period. In utero exposure to maternal smoking can methylate genes linked with cellular development and fetal growth, [34] cause fetal hypoxia [35] and alter hormone levels (e.g., leptin) that influence fetal (and possibly infantile) weight gain. In contrast, exposure to tobacco smoke during infancy can alter neurocircuitry for brain-to-gut communication, [36] alter infants' hormone levels, [37] and hypothalamic functions related to appetite control [24].

CAFFEINE

Prevalence and Sources of Intake

Caffeine is a naturally occurring alkaloid substance and a central nervous system stimulant present in food and beverages. It is one of the most commonly consumed dietary ingredients throughout the world and its consumption originates from ancient agricultural civilizations [38]. Caffeine is also produced synthetically and added to products (e.g., caffeinated sodas and energy drinks) to promote arousal, alertness, energy, and elevated mood. Caffeine is consumed by all population groups, including children and pregnant and lactating women [39, 40]. For example, during 2010–2011 in the United States, 43% of 2–5-year olds consumed caffeinated drinks; the proportion increased with age to almost 100% among those 65 and older [41]. Coffee is the single largest source of caffeine intake worldwide, followed by tea, caffeinated drinks, and chocolate [42]. The consumption of energy drinks is growing source of caffeine intake worldwide, particularly among adolescents and young adults. For example, from 2003 to 2006 in the United States, the prevalence of energy drink consumption increased from 0.5 to 5.5% among young adults [43]. In Norway, the sale of energy drinks increased by 60% from 2015 to 2018, and a total of 19%, 53%, and 70% of people in the age groups 10–12 years, 13–15 years, and 16–18 years, respectively, reported that they consumed energy drinks occasionally [44].

As high caffeine intake can be harmful, public health agencies have issued guidelines that limit daily caffeine intake according to age and life stage. Pregnant and breastfeeding women are advised to limit their caffeine intake as much as possible, with an upper limit of 200 mg daily considered safe [45]. However, it can be difficult to heed this advice because there is wide variation in individuals' sensitivity to the stimulating effects of caffeine, how fast caffeine is metabolized, and because caffeinated products vary widely in their caffeine content. For example, the caffeine content of coffee differs with brewing method and brand. An 8 oz cup of coffee is 80–100 mg of caffeine, compared with 30–50 mg in a typical cup of black tea, 30–40 mg in a can of caffeinated soda, and 40–250 mg in a can of energy drink [46].

Bioavailability

Caffeine is soluble in water and lipids and is present in all body fluids, including breast milk. Caffeine is an "antagonist" molecule: it binds to receptors located in the central and peripheral nervous systems, in blood vessels, and in various organs including the heart. Caffeine has multiple functions throughout the body and is particularly important for metabolic activity, cell signaling, and regulation [47].

After ingestion, caffeine is rapidly and completely absorbed in the gastrointestinal tract. Peak caffeine concentration in saliva occurs 45 minutes after ingestion and in plasma about two hours after ingestion [47]. Caffeine half-life depends on rate of elimination and varies with age, life-stage, genetics, and environmental factors [48]. In humans, caffeine is primarily (95%) metabolized in the liver by the CYP1A2 enzyme of the cytochrome P450 oxidase system. Tobacco smoke induces cytochrome CYP1A2 resulting in increased rate of caffeine metabolism and shortening the half-life of caffeine [48]. Caffeine half-life is 3–7 hours in non-pregnant adults and longer (up to 16 hours) during pregnancy; the half-life returns to baseline within the first week postpartum [48, 49].

Caffeine is rapidly transferred to the fetus during pregnancy and to breast milk, with peak concentration usually occurring approximately one hour after ingestion [50]. Among neonates, the half-life is even longer than in pregnant women—between 65 and 130 hours—due to neonates' immature kidneys and liver. Furthermore, caffeine elimination is slower in breastfed than in formula-fed infants [51]. The slower elimination rate among breastfed infants is important as the effects of caffeine depend on the peak concentration and length of time it remains in tissues [47]. Still, caffeine is not contraindicated for all infants. For example, the stimulant effect of caffeine has clinical applications for treatment of breathing problems (apnea) in very premature babies [52]. In light of the slow elimination of caffeine during early infancy, exposure through breast milk may pose harmful short and/or long-term effects on infant weight gain. However, the potential effects on caffeine exposure during the postnatal period on weight gain and growth is unknown.

Contrary to the knowledge gap as to the link between caffeine exposure through breast milk and infant weight gain and growth, in utero caffeine exposure has been linked to fetal growth restriction [47]. The putative biological mechanisms for fetal growth restriction and postnatal excess growth are provided by animal studies and include reduced placental blood flow [53] and genetic programming towards a thrifty phenotype [54]. In animal studies, prenatal caffeine exposure induces alteration in gene expression in the hypothalamic-pituitary-adrenocortical axis, which plays a key role in growth and metabolism [55–58]. Prenatal caffeine exposure may also alter regulation of adenosine and adenosine antagonists, which may modulate growth during infancy, [59, 60] and may induce alteration in the placental expression and transportation of leptin, [61] a hormone essential for appetite regulation.

Caffeine Exposure, Weight Gain, and Growth during Infancy and Childhood

Considering the widespread consumption of caffeine there are surprisingly few published studies on caffeine exposure through breast milk and its health effects during infancy and childhood. A systematic review of the evidence (published through October 2017) on the effects of maternal caffeine consumption on breastfed infants aged 0–6 months concluded that there was insufficient and inconsistent evidence on outcomes including 24-hour heart rate, 24-hour sleep time, and frequent night waking [62]. None of the identified studies examined infant growth or weight gain. However, two animal studies showed that rat pups either exposed to caffeine through injection [63] or through addition to the drinking water of lactating dams [64] grew more slowly during the lactation period than non-exposed pups. In the former study, pups were injected with 1 or 9 mg caffeine per kilogram in the first week of life. According to the authors, the two doses are equivalent to a 1/3 cup and 3 cups of coffee [63]. In the latter study, dams were given solutions resulting in morning milk caffeine concentrations in the range of 7–40 µg/ml, which is considerably higher than the mean caffeine concentration of 0.82 µg/ml in breast milk from 18 women sampled after habitual morning coffee consumption [65].

While prospective cohort studies on caffeine exposure through breastfeeding and growth during childhood are lacking, observational studies have reported robust associations between prenatal caffeine exposure and fetal growth restriction [47, 66, 67]. Four studies have reported adverse associations between maternal caffeine intake during pregnancy and offspring growth patterns during infancy and/or childhood through age 15 years [67–70]. Among 558 mother–infant pairs participating in the Lifeways Cross-Generation Cohort Study in Ireland (enrolled 2002), an increment of 100 µg/day of maternal caffeine intake was associated with a higher BMI z-score of 0.13 (95% CI: 0.06, 0.21) at 5 years and of 0.17 (95% CI: 0.04, 0.29) at 9 years old [68]. The corresponding increase in overall obesity were odds ratios of 1.32 (95% CI: 1.11, 1.60) at 5 years and 1.62 (95% CI: 1.12, 2.34) at 9 years old. Caffeine exposure of fathers and grandparents was not associated with offspring adiposity or obesity risk. Adjustment for breastfeeding duration did not influence the results.

Among 7,857 mother–infant participants in the Netherlands' Generation R pregnancy cohort (enrolled 2001–2005), compared to infants whose mothers consumed the equivalent of less than 2 cups of coffee per day (90 mg of caffeine), infants of mothers who consumed the equivalent of 4–5.9 cups and ≥6 cups of caffeine were shorter and had lower weights at birth, but gained more weight from birth to 6 years [69]. They tended to be shorter and to have higher body mass and total body fat mass. For example, the differences in total body fat mass z-scores between the two consumption groups were 0.10 (95% CI: 0.01, 0.20; $p < .05$) and 0.18 (95% CI: –0.01, 0.37; $p < .05$), respectively, at 6 years of age. The results were independent of infant feeding method.

Among 50,943 mother–child pairs in the Norwegian Mother and Child Cohort Study followed until the child aged 8 years old (enrolled 2002–2008), [67] prenatal caffeine exposure predicted excess infant growth, defined as a World Health Organization weight gain z-score of greater than 0.67 from birth to age 1 year, and with being overweight or obese, using the International Obesity Task Force criteria [71]. Compared with caffeine intake of <50 mg/day, caffeine intakes of 50–199 mg/day (44%), 200–299 mg/day (7%), and ≥300 mg/day (3%) predicted excess infant growth: adjusted ORs (aOR) of 1.15 (95% CI: 1.09, 1.22), 1.30 (95% CI: 1.16, 1.45), and 1.66 (95% CI: 1.42, 1.93), respectively. The corresponding risks of being overweight at 3 years old were 1.05 (95% CI: 0.99, 1.22), 1.17 (95% CI: 1.05, 1.30), and 1.44 (95% CI: 1.24, 1.67). Similar odds ratios were found at age 5, while at age 8, the risk was significant only for the highest caffeine intake category with an aOR of 1.29 (95% CI: 1.04, 1.66). Paternal caffeine intake did not predict offsprings' risk of excess growth or weight.

Among 829 mother–child pairs in a U.S. pregnancy cohort followed for 15 years (enrolled 1996–1998), [70] compared to children whose mothers did not consume caffeine during pregnancy, the odds ratio of childhood obesity was 1.77 (95% CI: 1.05, 3.00) for prenatal caffeine intake of <150 mg/day and 2.67 (1.24, 4.52) for prenatal caffeine intake of ≥150 mg/day. The results were adjusted for feeding method and a number of other potential confounding factors.

Self-reported breastfeeding was included among the confounding variables in three studies [68–70] and smoking was included among the confounding variables in all the above studies [67–70]. All studies reported that maternal smoking was associated with higher caffeine intake during pregnancy; there were no consistent findings concerning the association between caffeine intake and breastfeeding. None of the studies examined the associations between caffeine exposure during breastfeeding and growth or weight gain during infancy or childhood.

Timing of Exposure

Women who ingest caffeine during pregnancy will almost certainly also do so after pregnancy and the effect of caffeine exposure through breast milk should be accounted for in studies of in utero and postnatal caffeine exposure and weight gain during infancy and childhood. Intrauterine growth restriction will inherently affect catch-up growth in the first year of life [72]. The interaction of breastfeeding and a continuation of caffeine exposure in breastfed infants represents a knowledge gap. Whether caffeine ingested through breastfeeding further strengthens the adverse impact of prenatal caffeine or whether other components in breast milk counteract some of the negative programming effects is unknown. More studies are needed to assess the potential impact of caffeine exposure through breast milk on growth and weight gain during infancy and childhood.

CANNABIS

Prevalence and Sources of Intake

Due to its increasing legality and multiple forms, cannabis use is becoming more prevalent, even among those with children in the home [73]. According to United States' National Survey on Drug Use and Health (2016–2017), 7.0% of pregnant women aged 12–44 used cannabis in the "past month," an increase from 3.4% in 2002 [74]. According to the Pregnancy Risk Assessment Monitoring System, in Alaska and Vermont (2009–2011), two states where medical (but not recreational) cannabis use was legal during time of the survey, 6.8% of breastfeeding women used cannabis [75]. In Colorado (2014–2015), where recreational cannabis was (and is) legal, 5.0% of women who breastfed used cannabis within 4 months postpartum; of those that breastfed for less than 8 weeks, the prevalence was 10% [76]. Actual prevalence is likely to be higher. For example, among 279,457 pregnant women enrolled in Kaiser Permanente Northern California healthcare system (2009–2016) with positive cannabis toxicology tests administered at around 8 weeks' gestation during standard prenatal care, only 45% reported using cannabis on a self-administered questionnaire [77].

Bioavailability

The primary method for cannabis intake is inhalation of the smoke from dried cannabis sativa plants, through which both major cannabinoids, $\Delta 9$-tetrahydrocannabinol (THC) and cannabidiol (CBD), are ingested [78].

However, particularly as legalization becomes more widespread, products which contain THC, CBD, or both can be ingested in the form of vaping (in electronic cigarettes), food, pills and capsules, and skin oils and patches.

Given that cannabinoids are fat soluble, reliable estimation of its bioavailability in breast milk only became available in the 2010s [79–81]. In 54 breast milk samples from 50 cannabis users, modern testing methods detected THC up to 6 days after the last reported use (median 9.47ng/ml; range 1.01–323.00) [82]. Among a group of 8 women with a positive urine test for cannabis at labor and delivery who had abstained from cannabis use following childbirth, THC was still detectable in their milk at 6 weeks postpartum (median 1.7ng/ml; range 1.2–1.9) [83]. This study also found that THC continued to be detectable in breast milk after it was no longer detectable in plasma and urine.

While plasma bioavailability of THC after oral consumption by adults is only 6 ± 3% of the THC in the initial product, [84] plasma bioavailability after inhalation is 10 ± 7% among people who do not use more than once per month and 23 ± 16% among daily users [85]. Absorption and therefore peak plasma levels occur significantly more rapidly after inhalation, often within minutes, [86, 87] compared to 1–3 hours after oral consumption [84, 88, 89]. As a result, peak plasma levels are higher following inhalation at the same dose of cannabinoids. Likewise, cannabis metabolites differ in both amount and type after inhalation versus oral ingestion [84, 90, 91]. It is therefore possible that maternal ingestion method creates different toxicity profiles, especially if the degree of harm to a developing fetus or infant correlates with overall peak plasma levels and/or different metabolite exposures [92]. Similarly, the degree and type of harm to an infant may differ depending on whether they ingest cannabinoids through breast milk or secondhand smoke (SHS); although it seems likely that the latter would pose a greater risk due to the toxins in SHS (see below). To the best of our knowledge, there are no studies that determine whether the levels and types of cannabinoids transferred to breast milk vary by consumption route or specific cannabinoid(s) ingested.

The bioavailability of cannabinoids in infants following ingestion through breast milk has not been established. In one case report, THC metabolites in the infant's feces were in differing proportions to those in their mother's milk, therefore providing evidence that infants absorb and metabolize cannabinoids and do not merely excrete them [93]. Although an infant's plasma THC concentration is estimated to be approximately 1000-fold lower than the concentration in an adult, [82] THC is stored in fat tissue and eliminated at a slower rate than plasma [94]. There is therefore concern for the effects of the accumulation of cannabinoids and their metabolites in an infant exposed to cannabis, especially if those around the infant are frequent and/or heavy users.

Pathway

Cannabinoids may affect infant growth through several potential pathways. Low maternal milk supply can result in poor infant growth. In two double-blind, randomized studies, baseline prolactin (a hormone involved in milk supply) levels were significantly lower in frequent (≥ 10 cannabis exposures in the past month; N = 40) versus non-users (N = 36) of cannabis, [95] as well between heavy (≥ 3 cannabis cigarettes/day for ≥ 6 months; N = 12) and light/occasional (<3 cigarettes/day for ≥ 6 months; N = 11) users [96]. Animal studies have found prolactin reductions of between 85% and 90% within 30–90 minutes of THC administration [97, 98]. Other consequences of THC administration in lactating animals include a reduction in oxytocin release in response to suckling, leading to delayed milk ejection, lower milk consumption, lethargy, reduced maternal care, and anxiety [98–101]. These factors in combination can lead to considerably lower infant caloric intake.

Secondly, little is known about the contents of secondhand cannabis smoke or the byproducts of vaping THC. However, there is some evidence that cannabis smoke has the potential to affect growth in the same ways as secondhand tobacco smoke. Cannabis smoke has the same respiratory disease-causing carcinogenic chemicals as tobacco smoke, with some occurring in much higher quantities [102–104]. For example, one study found levels of ammonia 20 times higher and hydrogen cyanide, aromatic amines, and polycyclic aromatic hydrocarbons at concentrations 3–5 times higher than tobacco smoke [102]. In addition, given its continued illicit status in many jurisdictions, there is significantly less regulation and oversight of the pesticides, herbicides, rodenticides, and fertilizers used to grow cannabis, many of which are known toxins [105]. There is growing evidence that exposure to environmental contaminants such as these affects both fetal and infant growth [106].

Cannabis Exposure through Breastfeeding, Weight Gain and Growth during Infancy and Childhood

Most postpartum cannabis users also use while pregnant: among 68 mothers from Washington state (1982–1984) who had used cannabis during lactation, only 1 in 5 had not also used it during pregnancy [107]. Therefore, isolating the effects of cannabis use during breastfeeding while also controlling for confounding factors, such as alcohol and tobacco use during pregnancy, is difficult. Only one study has examined the specific effects of cannabis ingested through breast milk on growth [108].

Among a group of 756 predominantly "lower-middle to lower-class" (p. 49) residents of Denver, Colorado (1981–1982), the mean birth length of infants born to mothers who smoked an average of three cannabis cigarettes per day during the first trimester was .55 cm less, independent of confounding factors [108]. However, cannabis use did not predict birth weight, head circumference, or results of various newborn tests. In addition, maternal cannabis use during breastfeeding did not predict growth of the infants in this study. Of the 129 participants who were followed until age one, 27 had breastfed and used cannabis; there was no difference in growth (or mental or motor development) between infants of users and nonusers, even among those infants exposed to cannabis during pregnancy *and* breastfeeding.

Animal studies demonstrate that milk-fed offspring of both rhesus monkey [101] and mice [109] mothers administered cannabis/THC gain weight at a slower rate than an unexposed control group. The mouse pup treatment group had slower weight gain between days 4–15 and weighed 10–14% less than controls (treatment: 7.13 ± 0.24g; control: 8.30 ± 0.22; $p \leq .05$) at weaning (day 21) [109]. Given that other developmental milestones such as tail length and eye opening were not significantly affected, the researchers attributed their findings to malnutrition, perhaps because of poorer milk production or the influence of THC on the offspring. Infant rhesus monkeys who ingested THC through their mothers' milk took longer to regain their birth weight and had a slower rate of growth overall: only two out of five in the treatment group doubled their weight by five months, whereas all control group (N = 5) infants had [101]. Monkey mothers and offspring both appeared lethargic during feeding. Although the mean weights of the treatment groups were lower at monkey weaning (treatment: 884 ± 174g; control: 993 ± 121g), this difference was not statistically significant. While these findings suggest that long-term weight gain of mothers' milk-fed offspring is independent of maternal THC ingestion, it is important to note that the small sample size and two "particularly large and vigorously healthy" (p. 1080) [101] infants in the monkey treatment group may have contributed to this failure to achieve statistical significance. While animal studies may have limited applicability to humans, they nevertheless provide evidence of concerning behaviors and outcomes because of maternal cannabis consumption. Whether this is the case in humans is unknown given the absence of data on the long-term effects of maternal cannabis use during lactation alone.

Timing of Exposure

Cannabinoids readily cross the placenta [92, 101] and human cannabinoid receptors are active from 19 weeks of gestation [110]. The body's own endocannabinoid system, a cell-signaling system comprised of receptors that interpret cannabinoids both produced by the body and introduced into it, is involved in immunoregulation and neuroprotection [111]. Therefore, the introduction of external cannabinoids may affect appropriate fetal immune and neurological development: in early pregnancy, immune regulation is essential to fundamental gestation events such as decidualization (the process of changes in the endometrium in preparation for, and during, pregnancy), embryo implantation, and fetal development [111]. Cannabinoids can also affect fetal dopamine, opioid, GABA, glutamate, and serotonin-associated systems [112] and therefore later eating, satiety, and growth patterns.

Data on more immediate effects of prenatal exposure on fetal growth and obstetric outcomes conflict [113]. A meta-analysis found that prenatal cannabis use predicts elevated odds of prenatal maternal anemia (pooled OR (pOR) 1.36; 95% CI: 1.10, 1.69; $p < .005$), decreased birth weight (1.77; 1.04, 3.01; $p < .05$; pooled mean difference 109.42g; 38.72–180.12g; $p < .005$), and a higher likelihood of neonatal intensive care (NICU) admission (pOR 2.02; 1.27, 3.21; $p < .005$), [114] which increases the likelihood of interrupted or non-initiation of breastfeeding [115]. However, after controlling for prenatal tobacco use and socioeconomic and demographic factors, a second meta-analysis did not find any statistically significant associations between cannabis use and any adverse neonatal outcomes [116].

Other studies—not included in these meta-analyses—nevertheless continue to find associations between prenatal cannabis use and adverse neonatal outcomes. For example, among 1,610 singleton births (United States; 2006–2008) and after controlling for tobacco use and socioeconomic factors, maternal cannabis use predicted an elevated risk for neonatal morbidity or death (14.1% in users, 4.5% in non-users; aOR 3.11; 95% CI: 1.40, 6.91; $p = .002$), especially infections (9.8% vs. 2.4%; $p < .001$) and neurological conditions (1.4% vs. 0.3%; $p = .002$) [117]. Among 5,588 nulliparous participants with singleton pregnancies (Australia, New Zealand, Ireland, and United Kingdom; 2004–2011) after controlling for maternal age, cigarette smoking, alcohol and socioeconomic factors, continued prenatal cannabis use at 20 weeks' gestation was associated with over five-fold increase in the risk of spontaneous preterm birth (aOR 5.44; 95% CI: 2.44, 12.11; $p < .001$) [118]. Among 243,140 pregnant women (Canada, 2008–2016) found an elevated risk of SGA (aOR 1.47; 95% CI: 1.33, 1.61, $p < .0001$), spontaneous preterm birth (aOR 1.27; 95% CI: 1.14, 1.42; $p < .01$) and intrapartum stillbirth (adjusted hazard ratio 2.84; 95% CI: 1.18, 6.82; $p < .02$) independently of maternal age, pre-pregnancy body mass index, tobacco use, alcohol use, other substance use, socioeconomic status, and race/ethnicity [119]. A matched cohort study of 98,512 women (Canada, 2012–2017), self-reported prenatal cannabis use was significantly associated with, among others, preterm birth (RR 1.41; 95% CI: 1.25–1.47), SGA (RR 1.53; 95% CI: 1.45, 1.61), and [120].

Longitudinal studies, such as the Ottawa Prenatal Prospective Study (N = 190; Canada; enrolled 1978; growth data up to 18 years old) and Maternal Health Practices and Child Development Project (N = 763; United States; enrolled 1982–1985; growth data up to 6 years old), have not found that prenatal cannabis use affects long-term physical growth [92]. The Ottawa Prenatal Prospective Study also did not find any differences in key pubertal milestones, such as menstruation in females and shaving in males [121, 122]. Nevertheless, these and other longitudinal studies have found a variety of poorer neurological, psychological, and developmental outcomes, such as decreased attention, impulse control, and verbal/memory processing and increased depression, anxiety, and hyperactivity [92].

Prenatal cannabis use may, however, protect against the occurrence of large gestational age (LGA) when there are maternal risk factors. LGA newborns have a higher risk of later obesity: in one study (United States; 2009–2017), they were twice as likely to be overweight/obese at preschool age (4–6 years old) (OR 2.01; 95% CI: 1.90, 2.13; $p < .01$) [123]. These odds increase to 2.79 (2.35, 3.30; $p < .01$) for LGA newborns of mothers with gestational diabetes. In a retrospective cohort study (United States; 2012–2016) of 298 pregnant women with either gestational or pre-existing diabetes, the 38 (13%) that used cannabis were 78% less likely to have LGA newborns (5.3% versus 19%; aOR 0.22; 0.05, 0.98) after controlling for tobacco use [124].

CONCLUSION

Evidence suggests that exposure to substance through breast milk can influence the rate of weight gain and growth during infancy. Prime examples include use of nicotine, caffeine, and cannabis use during the postnatal period. However, research has predominantly focused on use during pregnancy, largely ignoring the effect on an infant due to exposure through breast milk. Animal studies provide indications that there may be detrimental effects from exposure to these substances through maternal milk, but even this data is scant. Other potentially important interacting maternal influences include variables pertaining to pregnancy, such as the amount of gestational weight gain, [126] and the many other maternal behaviors that influence biological and physiological determinants of rate of weight gain and growth during infancy [127]. With breastfeeding rates increasing internationally, the need to study the effects on offspring of substances transferred into breast milk is ever more pressing. This information can also inform future interventions. For example, a primary intervention can be through enhanced maternal prenatal and postpartum nutrition, one of the few maternal interventions with documented improvements in fetal and postnatal growth. In this instance, guidelines for postpartum nutrition can be modified to account for smoking status, caffeine intake, and cannabis use.

On a practical note, those feeding breast milk, their own or donated, to infants in their care may ask their healthcare professionals for advice about these—and other—substances in that milk. For most substances, complete abstinence may not be practical nor warranted, given that the existing, albeit limited, data seem to suggest a dose response. Healthcare professionals need to provide accurate, realistic, non-judgmental information while educating about risks to both the breastfeeder and those consuming their milk. When counseling a caregiver, professionals should also acknowledge actual or perceived benefits—emotional, social—to using these substances. Allowing for an honest dialogue is not only best practice, but also creates an environment where a caregiver may more honestly disclose the use of substances, perhaps even substances more detrimental than those discussed in this chapter.

REFERENCES

[1] Gillman MW, Ludwig DS. How early should obesity prevention start? *New Engl J Medicine.* 2013;369(23):2173-2175. doi:10.1056/nejmp1310577.

[2] Gillman MW, Rifas-Shiman SL, Kleinman K, Oken E, Rich-Edwards JW, Taveras EM. Developmental origins of childhood overweight: Potential public health impact. *Obesity.* 2008;16(7): 1651-1656. doi:10.1038/oby.2008.260.

[3] Stettler N. Nature and strength of epidemiological evidence for origins of childhood and adulthood obesity in the first year of life. *Int J Obesity.* 2007;31(7):1035-1043. doi:10.1038/sj.ijo.0803659.

[4] Monteiro P, Victora C. Rapid growth in infancy and childhood and obesity in later life—a systematic review. *Obes Rev.* 2005;6(2):143-154. doi:10.1111/j.1467-789x.2005.00183.x.

[5] Gardner DS, Hosking J, Metcalf BS, Jeffery AN, Voss LD, Wilkin TJ. Contribution of early weight gain to childhood overweight and metabolic health: a longitudinal study (EarlyBird 36). *Pediatrics.* 2009;123(1):e67-73. doi:10.1542/peds.2008-1292.

[6] Dennison BA, Edmunds LS, Stratton HH, Pruzek RM. Rapid infant weight gain predicts childhood overweight. *Obesity.* 2006;14(3):491-499. doi:10.1038/oby.2006.64.

[7] Curtin SC, Matthews T. Smoking prevalence and cessation before and during pregnancy: Data from the birth certificate, 2014. *Natl Vital Stat Rep.* 2016;65(1):1-14.

[8] Livingstone-Banks J, Norris E, Hartmann-Boyce J, West R, Jarvis M, Hajek P. Relapse prevention interventions for smoking cessation. *Cochrane Db Syst Rev.* 2019;2(2):CD003999. doi:10.1002/14651858.cd003999.pub5.

[9] Chamberlain C, O'Mara-Eves A, Porter J, et al. Psychosocial interventions for supporting women to stop smoking in pregnancy. *Cochrane Db Syst Rev*. 2017;2(2):CD001055. doi:10.1002/14651 858.cd001055.pub5.

[10] Quickstats: Smoking cessation* during pregnancy — 46 states and the District of Columbia, 2014. *MMWR*. 2016;65(22):588. doi:10. 15585/mmwr.mm6522a6.

[11] Pollak KI, Oncken CA, Lipkus IM, et al. Nicotine replacement and behavioral therapy for smoking cessation in pregnancy. *Am J Prev Med*. 2007;33(4):297-305. doi:10.1016/j.amepre.2007.05.006.

[12] Hotham ED, Gilbert AL, Atkinson ER. A randomised-controlled pilot study using nicotine patches with pregnant women. *Addict Behav*. 2006;31(4):641-648. doi:10.1016/j.addbeh.2005.05.042.

[13] Myung S-K, Ju W, Jung H-S, et al. Efficacy and safety of pharmacotherapy for smoking cessation among pregnant smokers: A meta-analysis. *BJOG*. 2012;119(9):1029-1039. doi:10.1111/j.1471-0528.2012.03408.x.

[14] Smedberg J, Lupattelli A, Mårdby AC, Nordeng H. Characteristics of women who continue smoking during pregnancy: A cross-sectional study of pregnant women and new mothers in 15 European countries. *BMC Pregnancy Childb*. 2014;14(1):213. doi:10.1186/ 1471-2393-14-213.

[15] Haidar YM, Cosman BC. Obesity epidemiology. *Clin Colon Rect Surg*. 2011;24(4):205-210. doi:10.1055/s-0031-1295684.

[16] Hellström-Lindahl E, Court J. Nicotinic acetylcholine receptors during prenatal development and brain pathology in human aging. *Behav Brain Res*. 2000;113(1-2):159-168. doi:10.1016/s0166-4328 (00)00210-2.

[17] Slotkin TA. If nicotine is a developmental neurotoxicant in animal studies, dare we recommend nicotine replacement therapy in pregnant women and adolescents? *Neurotoxicol Teratol*. 2008; 30(1):1-19. doi:10.1016/j.ntt.2007.09.002.

[18] Dahlström A, Ebersjö C, Lundell B. Nicotine exposure in breastfed infants. *Acta Paediatr.* 2004;93(6):810-816. doi:10.1111/j.1651-2227.2004.tb03023.x.

[19] Schulte-Hobein B, Schwartz-Bickenbach D, Abt S, Plum C, Nau H. Cigarette smoke exposure and development of infants throughout the first year of life: Influence of passive smoking and nursing on cotinine levels in breast milk and infant's urine. *Acta Paediatr.* 1992;81(6-7):550-557. doi:10.1111/j.1651-2227.1992.tb12293.x.

[20] Oken E, Levitan E, Gillman M. Maternal smoking during pregnancy and child overweight: systematic review and meta-analysis. *Int J Obesity.* 2008;32(2):201-210. doi:10.1038/sj.ijo.0803760.

[21] Ong KK, Loos RJ. Rapid infancy weight gain and subsequent obesity: Systematic reviews and hopeful suggestions. *Acta Paediatr.* 2006;95(8):904-908. doi:10.1080/08035250600719754.

[22] Szlagatys-Sidorkiewicz A, Martysiak-Żurowska D, Krzykowski G, Zagierski M, Kamińska B. Maternal smoking modulates fatty acid profile of breast milk. *Acta Paediatr.* 2013;102(8):e353-e359. doi: 10.1111/apa.12276.

[23] Much D, Brunner S, Vollhardt C, et al. Breast milk fatty acid profile in relation to infant growth and body composition: results from the INFAT study. *Pediatr Res.* 2013;74(2):230. doi:10.1038/pr.2013.82.

[24] Jo Y-H, Talmage DA, Role LW. Nicotinic receptor-mediated effects on appetite and food intake. *J Neurobiol.* 2002;53(4):618-632. doi:10.1002/neu.10147.

[25] Coutant R, de Casson BF, Douay O, et al. Relationships between placental GH concentration and maternal smoking, newborn gender, and maternal leptin: Possible implications for birth weight. *J Clin Endocrinol Metabolism.* 2001;86(10):4854-4859. doi:10.1210/jcem.86.10.7971.

[26] Williamson D, Madans J, Anda R, Kleinman J, Giovino G, Byers T. Smoking cessation and severity of weight gain in a national cohort. *New Engl J Medicine.* 1991;324(11):739-745. doi:10.1056/nejm199103143241106.

[27] Moore B, Sauder K, Starling A, Ringham B, Glueck D, Dabelea D. Exposure to secondhand smoke, exclusive breastfeeding and infant adiposity at age 5 months in the Healthy Start study. *Pediatr Obes.* 2017;12 Suppl 1(S1):111-119. doi:10.1111/ijpo.12233.

[28] Little R, Lambert, Worthington-Roberts B, Ervin C. Maternal smoking during lactation: Relation to infant size at one year of age. *Am J Epidemiol.* 1994;140(6):544-554. doi:10.1093/oxfordjournals.aje.a117281.

[29] Boshuizen H, Verkerk P, Reerink J, Herngreen W, Zaadstra B, Verloove-Vanhorick S. Maternal smoking during lactation: Relation to growth during the first year of life in a Dutch birth cohort. *Am J Epidemiol.* 1998;147(2):117-126. doi:10.1093/oxfordjournals.aje.a009423.

[30] Shenassa ED, Wen X, Braid S. Exposure to tobacco metabolites via breast milk and infant weight gain: A population-based study. *J Hum Lact.* 2016;32(3):462-471. doi:10.1177/0890334415619154.

[31] Taal HR, vander Heijden AJ, Steegers EA, Hofman A, Jaddoe VW. Small and large size for gestational age at birth, infant growth, and childhood overweight. *Obesity.* 2013;21(6):1261-1268. doi:10.1002/oby.20116.

[32] Shenassa ED. Maternal smoking during pregnancy and offspring weight gain: A consideration of competing explanations. *Paediatr Perinat Ep.* 2017;31(5):409-411. doi:10.1111/ppe.12405.

[33] Pattenden S, Antova T, Neuberger M, et al. Parental smoking and children's respiratory health: Independent effects of prenatal and postnatal exposure. *Tob Control.* 2006;15(4):294. doi:10.1136/tc.2005.015065.

[34] Küpers LK, Xu X, Jankipersadsing SA, et al. DNA methylation mediates the effect of maternal smoking during pregnancy on birthweight of the offspring. *Int J Epidemiol.* 2015;44(4):1224-1237. doi:10.1093/ije/dyv048.

[35] Khuc K, Blanco E, Burrows R, et al. Adolescent metabolic syndrome risk is increased with higher infancy weight gain and

decreased with longer breast feeding. *Int J Pediatrics.* 2012;2012 (4):478610. doi:10.1155/2012/478610.

[36] Pray LA, and Board F, of Medicine I. *Examining a Developmental Approach to Childhood Obesity: The Fetal and Early Childhood Years: Workshop Summary.* Washington, D.C.: National Academies Press; 2015. doi:10.17226/21782.

[37] Eliasson B, Smith U. Leptin levels in smokers and long-term users of nicotine gum. *Eur J Clin Invest.* 1999;29(2):145-152. doi:10.1046/j. 1365-2362.1999.00420.x.

[38] Lachance MP. The pharmacology and toxicology of caffeine. *J Food Safety.* 1982;4(2):71-112. doi:10.1111/j.1745-4565.1982.tb00435.x.

[39] Ahluwalia N, Herrick K. *Caffeine intake from food and beverage sources and trends among children and adolescents in the United States: Review of national quantitative studies from 1999 to 2011. Adv Nutr.* 2015;6(1):102-111. doi:10.3945/an.114.007401.

[40] Heckman MA, Weil J, de Mejia E. Caffeine (1, 3, 7-trimethylxanthine) in foods: A comprehensive review on consumption, functionality, safety, and regulatory matters. *J Food Sci.* 2010;75(3):R77 R87. doi:10.1111/j.1750-3841.2010.01561.x.

[41] Mitchell DC, Knight CA, Hockenberry J, Teplansky R, Hartman TJ. Beverage caffeine intakes in the U.S. *Food Chem Toxicol.* 2014; 63:136-142. doi:10.1016/j.fct.2013.10.042.

[42] Verster JC, Koenig J. Caffeine intake and its sources: A review of national representative studies. *Crit Rev Food Sci.* 2018;58(8):1250-1259. doi:10.1080/10408398.2016.1247252.

[43] Vercammen KA, Koma WJ, Bleich SN. Trends in Energy Drink Consumption among U.S. Adolescents and Adults, 2003-2016. *Am J Prev Med.* 2019;56(6):827 833. doi:10.1016/j.amepre.2018.12.007.

[44] Iversen K, Arnesen E, Meltzer H, Brantsæter A. Children and adolescents need protection against energy drinks. *Tidsskrift Den Norske Legeforening.* 2018;138(14). doi:10.4045/tidsskr.18.0585.

[45] EFSA Panel on Dietetic Products, Nutrition and Allergies (NDA). Scientific opinion on the safety of caffeine. *EFSA J.* 2015;13(5): 4102. doi:10.2903/j.efsa.2015.4102.

[46] U.S. Food and Drug Administration. Spilling the Beans: How Much Caffeine is Too Much? https://www.fda.gov/consumers/consumer-updates/spilling-beans-how-much-caffeine-too-much. Published December 12, 2018. Accessed August 25, 2019.

[47] Temple JL, Bernard C, Lipshultz SE, Czachor JD, Westphal JA, Mestre MA. The safety of ingested caffeine: A comprehensive review. *Front Psychiatry.* 2017;8:80. doi:10.3389/fpsyt.2017.00080.

[48] Nehlig A. Interindividual differences in caffeine metabolism and factors driving caffeine consumption. *Pharmacol Rev.* 2018; 70(2):384-411. doi:10.1124/pr.117.014407.

[49] Knutti R, Rothweiler H, Schlatter C. The effect of pregnancy on the pharmacokinetics of caffeine. *Arch Toxicol.* 1982;5:187-192.

[50] U.S. National Library of Medicine. Caffeine. *Drugs and Lactation Database LactMed.* https://www.ncbi.nlm.nih.gov/books/NBK50 1467/. Published June 30, 2019. Accessed September 25, 2019.

[51] Guennec LJ, Billon B. Delay in caffeine elimination in breast-fed infants. *Pediatrics.* 1987;79(2):264-268.

[52] Abdel-Hady H, Nasef N, Shabaan A, Nour I. Caffeine therapy in preterm infants. *World J Clin Pediatrics.* 2015;4(4):81-93. doi:10. 5409/wjcp.v4.i4.81.

[53] Kirkinen P, Jouppila P, Koivula A, Vuori J, Puukka M. The effect of caffeine on placental and fetal blood flow in human pregnancy. *Am J Obstet Gynecol.* 1983;147(8):939-942. doi:10.1016/0002-9378(83) 90250-8.

[54] Wells JC. The thrifty phenotype: An adaptation in growth or metabolism? *Am J Hum Biol.* 2011;23(1):65-75. doi:10.1002/ajhb. 21100.

[55] Xu D, Wu Y, Liu F, et al. A hypothalamic-pituitary-adrenal axis-associated neuroendocrine metabolic programmed alteration in offspring rats of IUGR induced by prenatal caffeine ingestion.

Toxicol Appl Pharm. 2012;264(3):395-403. doi:10.1016/j.taap.2012. 08.016.

[56] Xu D, Zhang B, Liang G, et al. Caffeine-induced activated glucocorticoid metabolism in the hippocampus causes hypothalamic-pituitary-adrenal axis inhibition in fetal rats. *PloS One.* 2012;7(9):e44497. doi:10.1371/journal.pone.0044497.

[57] Li J, Luo H, Wu Y, et al. Gender-specific increase in susceptibility to metabolic syndrome of offspring rats after prenatal caffeine exposure with post-weaning high-fat diet. *Toxicol Appl Pharm.* 2015;284(3):345-353. doi:10.1016/j.taap.2015.03.002.

[58] He B, Wen Y, Hu S, et al. Prenatal caffeine exposure induces liver developmental dysfunction in offspring rats. *J Endocrinol.* 2019;242(3):211 226. doi:10.1530/joe-19-0066.

[59] Rivkees SA, Wendler CC. Adverse and protective influences of adenosine on the newborn and embryo: Implications for preterm white matter injury and embryo protection. *Pediatr Res.* 2011;69(4):271-278. doi:10.1203/pdr.0b013e31820efbcf.

[60] Buscariollo DL, Fang X, Greenwood V, Xue H, Rivkees SA, Wendler CC. Embryonic caffeine exposure acts via A1 adenosine receptors to alter adult cardiac function and DNA methylation in mice. *PloS One.* 2014;9(1):e87547. doi:10.1371/journal.pone. 0087547.

[61] Wu Y-M, Luo H-W, Kou H, et al. Prenatal caffeine exposure induced a lower level of fetal blood leptin mainly via placental mechanism. *Toxicol Appl Pharm.* 2015;289(1):109-116. doi:10. 1016/j.taap.2015.09.007.

[62] McCreedy A, Bird S, Brown LJ, Shaw-Stewart J, Chen Y-F. Effects of maternal caffeine consumption on the breastfed child: A systematic review. *Swiss Med Wkly.* 2018;148:w14665. doi:10.4414/smw.2018.14665.

[63] Zimmerberg B, Carr K, Scott A, Lee H, Weider J. The effects of postnatal caffeine exposure on growth, activity and learning in rats. *Pharmacol Biochem Be.* 1991;39(4):883-888. doi:10.1016/0091-3057(91)90048-7.

[64] Gullberg EI, Ferrell F, Christensen DH. Effects of postnatal caffeine exposure through dam's milk upon weanling rats. *Pharmacol Biochem Be*. 1986;24(6):1695 1701. doi:10.1016/0091-3057(86) 90507-1.

[65] Hildebrandt R, Gundert-Remy U. Lack of pharmacological active saliva levels of caffeine in breast-fed infants. *Pediatric pharmacology (New York, NY)*. 1983;3(3-4):237 244.

[66] Sengpiel V, Elind E, Bacelis J, et al. Maternal caffeine intake during pregnancy is associated with birth weight but not with gestational length: Results from a large prospective observational cohort study. *BMC Med*. 2013;11(1):42. doi:10.1186/1741-7015-11-42.

[67] Papadopoulou E, Botton J, Brantsæter A, et al. Maternal caffeine intake during pregnancy and childhood growth and overweight: Results from a large Norwegian prospective observational cohort study. *BMJ Open*. 2018;8(3):e018895. doi:10.1136/bmjopen-2017-018895.

[68] Chen L-W, Murrin CM, Mehegan J, Kelleher CC, Phillips CM, Cross-Generation Cohort Study for the Lifeways. Maternal, but not paternal or grandparental, caffeine intake is associated with childhood obesity and adiposity: The Lifeways Cross-Generation Cohort Study. *Am J Clin Nutrition*. 2019;109(6):1648-1655. doi:10.1093/ajcn/nqz019.

[69] Voerman E, Jaddoe VW, Gishti O, Hofman A, Franco OH, Gaillard R. Maternal caffeine intake during pregnancy, early growth, and body fat distribution at school age. *Obesity*. 2016;24(5):1170-1177. doi:10.1002/oby.21466.

[70] Li D, Ferber J, Odouli R. Maternal caffeine intake during pregnancy and risk of obesity in offspring: a prospective cohort study. *Int J Obesity*. 2015;39(4):658-664. doi:10.1038/ijo.2014.196.

[71] Cole TJ, Bellizzi MC, Flegal KM, Dietz WH. Establishing a standard definition for child overweight and obesity worldwide: International survey. *BMJ*. 2000;320(7244):1240. doi:10.1136/bmj.320.7244.1240.

[72] Osrin D, de Costello AM. What can be done about intrauterine growth retardation? *Seminars Neonatol.* 1999;4(3):173-181. doi:10.1016/s1084-2756(99)90050-7.

[73] Goodwin RD, Cheslack-Postava K, Santoscoy S, et al. Trends in Cannabis and Cigarette Use Among Parents With Children at Home: 2002 to 2015. *Pediatrics.* 2018;141(6):e20173506. doi:10.1542/peds. 2017-3506.

[74] Volkow ND, Han B, Compton WM, McCance-Katz EF. Self-reported Medical and Nonmedical Cannabis Use Among Pregnant Women in the United States. *JAMA.* 2019;322(2):167-169. doi:10.1001/jama.2019.7982.

[75] Ko JY, Tong VT, Bombard JM, Hayes DK, Davy J, Perham-Hester KA. Marijuana use during and after pregnancy and association of prenatal use on birth outcomes: A population-based study. *Drug Alcohol Depen.* 2018;187:72-78. doi:10.1016/j.drugalcdep.2018.02.017.

[76] Crume TL, Juhl AL, Brooks-Russell A, Hall KE, Wymore E, Borgelt LM. Cannabis use during the perinatal period in a state with legalized recreational and medical marijuana: The association between maternal characteristics, breastfeeding patterns, and neonatal outcomes. *J Pediatrics.* 2018;197:90-96. doi:10.1016/j.jpeds.2018.02.005.

[77] Young-Wolff KC, Tucker L-Y, Alexeeff S, et al. Trends in self-reported and biochemically tested marijuana use among pregnant females in California from 2009-2016. *JAMA.* 2017;318(24):2490-2491. doi:10.1001/jama.2017.17225.

[78] Grotenhermen F. Pharmacokinetics and pharmacodynamics of cannabinoids. *Clin Pharmacokinet.* 2003;42(4):327-360. doi:10.2165/00003088-200342040-00003.

[79] de Silveira G, Loddi S, de Oliveira C, Zucoloto A, Fruchtengarten L, Yonamine M. Headspace solid-phase microextraction and gas chromatography–mass spectrometry for determination of cannabinoids in human breast milk. *Forensic Toxicol.* 2016;35(1):125-132. doi:10.1007/s11419-016-0346-5.

[80] Anderson PO. Cannabis and breastfeeding. *Breastfeed Med.* 2017; 12(10):580-581. doi:10.1089/bfm.2017.0162.

[81] Wei B, McGuffey JE, Blount BC, Wang L. Sensitive quantification of cannabinoids in milk by alkaline saponification–solid phase extraction combined with isotope dilution UPLC–MS/MS. *Acs Omega.* 2016;1(6):1307-1313. doi:10.1021/acsomega.6b00253.

[82] Bertrand KA, Hanan NJ, Honerkamp-Smith G, Best BM, Chambers CD. Marijuana use by breastfeeding mothers and cannabinoid concentrations in breast milk. *Pediatrics.* 2018;142(3):e20181076. doi:10.1542/peds.2018-1076.

[83] Wymore E, Bunik M, Levek C, et al. Duration of marijuana excretion in human breast milk. *Breastfeed Med.* 2018;13(S2):S 40-S-41. doi:10.1089/bfm.2018.29106.abstracts.

[84] Ohlsson A, Lindgren J, Wahlen A, Agurell S, Hollister L, Gillespie H. Plasma delta-9-Tetrahydrocannabinol concentrations and clinical effects after oral and intravenous administration and smoking. *Clin Pharmacol Ther.* 1980;28(3):409-416. doi:10.1038/clpt.1980.181.

[85] Lindgren J-E, Ohlsson A, Agurell S, Hollister L, Gillespie H. Clinical effects and plasma levels of Δ9-Tetrahydrocannabinol (Δ9-THC) in heavy and light users of cannabis. *Psychopharmacology.* 1981;74(3):208-212. doi:10.1007/bf00427095.

[86] Kauert G, Ramaekers J, Schneider E, Moeller MR, Toennes SW. Pharmacokinetic properties of Δ9-Tetrahydrocannabinol in serum and oral fluid. *Endocrinology.* 2007;31:288-293. doi:10.1093/jat/31.5.288.

[87] Marsot A, Audebert C, Attolini L, Lacarelle B, Micallef J, Blin O. Comparison of cannabinoid concentrations in plasma, oral fluid and urine in occasional cannabis smokers after smoking cannabis cigarette. *J Pharm Pharm Sci.* 2016;19(3):411-422. doi:10.18433/j3f31d.

[88] Ahmed AI, van den Elsen GA, Colbers A, et al. Safety, pharmacodynamics, and pharmacokinetics of multiple oral doses of delta-9-tetrahydrocannabinol in older persons with dementia.

Psychopharmacology. 2015;232(14):2587-2595. doi:10.1007/s00213-015-3889-y.

[89] Schwilke EW, hwope D, Karschner EL, et al. Δ9-Tetrahydrocannabinol (THC), 11-Hydroxy-THC, and 11-Nor-9-carboxy-THC plasma pharmacokinetics during and after continuous high-dose oral THC. *Clin Chem*. 2009;55(12):2180-2189. doi:10.1373/clinchem.2008.122119.

[90] Newmeyer MN, Swortwood MJ, Barnes AJ, Abulseoud OA, Scheidweiler KB, Huestis MA. Free and glucuronide whole blood cannabinoids' pharmacokinetics after controlled smoked, vaporized, and oral cannabis administration in frequent and occasional cannabis users: Identification of recent cannabis intake. *Clin Chem*. 2016;62(12):1579-1592. doi:10.1373/clinchem.2016.263475.

[91] Huestis MA, Blount BC, Milan DF, Newmeyer MN, Schroeder J, Smith ML. Correlation of creatinine- and specific gravity-normalized free and glucuronidated urine cannabinoid concentrations following smoked, vaporized, and oral cannabis in frequent and occasional cannabis users. *Drug Test Anal*. 2019;11(7):968-975. doi:10.1002/dta.2576.

[92] Grant KS, Petroff R, Isoherranen N, Stella N, Burbacher TM. Cannabis use during pregnancy: Pharmacokinetics and effects on child development. *Pharmacol Therapeut*. 2018;182:133-151. doi:10.1016/j.pharmthera.2017.08.014.

[93] Perez-Reyes M, Wall ME. Presence of Δ9-tetrahydrocannabinol in human milk. *General Pharmacology*. 1982;307(13):819-820.

[94] Huestis MA. Human cannabinoid pharmacokinetics. *Chem Biodivers*. 2007;4(8):1770-1804. doi:10.1002/cbdv.200790152.

[95] Ranganathan M, Braley G, Pittman B, et al. The effects of cannabinoids on serum cortisol and prolactin in humans. *Psychopharmacology*. 2008;203(4):737-744. doi:10.1007/s00213-008-1422-2.

[96] x E, Pilotte NS, Adler WH, Nagel JE, Lange RW. The effects of 9-ene-tetrahydrocannabinol on hormone release and immune function.

J Steroid Biochemist. 1989;34(1-6):263-270. doi:10.1016/0022-4731 (89)90090-3.

[97] Asch RH, Smith CG, ler-Khodr T, Pauerstein CJ. Acute decreases in serum prolactin concentrations caused by Δ9-Tetrahydrocannabinol in nonhuman primates. *Fertil Steril*. 1979;32(5):571-575. doi:10.1016/s0015-0282(16)44362-1.

[98] Bromley B, Rabii J, Gordon J, Zimmermann E. Delta-9-Tetrahydrocannabinol inhibition of suckling-induced prolactin release in the lactating rat. *Endocr Res Commun*. 2009;5(4):271-278. doi:10.1080/07435807809061092.

[99] Tyrey L, Murphy LL. Inhibition of suckling-induced milk ejections in the lactating rat by Δ9-Tetrahydrocannabinol. *Endocrinology*. 1988;123(1):469-472. doi:10.1210/endo-123-1-469.

[100] Vilela FC, Giusti-Paiva A. Cannabinoid receptor agonist disrupts behavioral and neuroendocrine responses during lactation. *Behav Brain Res*. 2014;263:190-197. doi:10.1016/j.bbr.2014.01.037.

[101] Asch R, Smith C. Effects of delta 9-THC, the principal psychoactive component of marijuana, during pregnancy in the rhesus monkey. *The Journal of Reproductive Medicine*. 1986;31(12):1071-1081.

[102] Moir D, Rickert WS, Levasseur G, et al. A comparison of mainstream and sidestream marijuana and tobacco cigarette smoke produced under two machine smoking conditions. *Chem Res Toxicol*. 2008;21(2):494-502. doi:10.1021/tx700275p.

[103] Lee M, Novotny M, Bartle K. Gas chromatography/mass spectrometric and nuclear magnetic resonance spectrometric studies of carcinogenic polynuclear aromatic hydrocarbons in tobacco and marijuana smoke condensates. *Anal Chem*. 1976;48(2):405-416. doi:10.1021/ac60366a048.

[104] Rickert W, Robinson J, Rogers B. A comparison of tar, carbon monoxide and pH levels in smoke from marihuana and tobacco cigarettes. *Can J of Public Health*. 1982;73(6):386-391.

[105] Ryan SA, Ammerman SD, O'Connor ME, Committee on Substance Use and Prevention, Section on Breastfeeding. Marijuana Use During Pregnancy and Breastfeeding: Implications for Neonatal and

Childhood Outcomes. *Pediatrics.* 2018;142(3):e20181889. doi:10. 1542/peds.2018-1889.

[106] Kadawathagedara M, de Lauzon-Guillain B, Botton J. Environmental contaminants and child's growth. *J Dev Orig Hlth Dis.* 2018;9(6):632-641. doi:10.1017/s2040174418000995.

[107] Astley SJ, Little RE. Maternal marijuana use during lactation and infant development at one year. *Neurotoxicol Teratol.* 1990; 12(2):161-168. doi:10.1016/0892-0362(90)90129-z.

[108] Tennes K, Avitable N, Blackard C, et al. Marijuana: Prenatal and postnatal exposure in the human. *NIDA Research Monograph.* 1985;59:48-60.

[109] Frischknecht H, Sieber B, Waser P. The feeding of hashish to lactating mice: Effects on the development of sucklings. *General Pharmacology.* 1980;11(5):469-472.

[110] Mato S, Olmo E, Pazos A. Ontogenetic development of cannabinoid receptor expression and signal transduction functionality in the human brain. *Eur J Neurosci.* 2003;17(9):1747-1754. doi:10.1046/ j.1460-9568.2003.02599.x.

[111] Fride E. Multiple roles for the endocannabinoid system during the earliest stages of life: Pre- and postnatal development. *J Neuroendocrinol.* 2008;20(s1):75-81. doi:10.1111/j.1365-2826.2008. 01670.x.

[112] Jutras-Aswad D, DiNieri JA, Harkany T, Hurd YL. Neurobiological consequences of maternal cannabis on human fetal development and its neuropsychiatric outcome. *Eur Arch Psy Clin N.* 2009;259(7):395-412. doi:10.1007/s00406-009-0027-z.

[113] Stickrath E. Marijuana use in pregnancy: An updated look at marijuana use and its impact on pregnancy. *Clin Obstet Gynecol.* 2019;62(1):185-190. doi:10.1097/grf.0000000000000415.

[114] Gunn J, Rosales C, Center K, et al. Prenatal exposure to cannabis and maternal and child health outcomes: A systematic review and meta-analysis. *BMJ Open.* 2016;6(4):e009986. doi:10.1136/ bmjopen-2015-009986.

[115] Gertz B, DeFranco E. Predictors of breastfeeding non-initiation in the NICU. *Maternal Child Nutrition.* 2019;15(3):e12797. doi:10.1111/ mcn.12797.

[116] Conner SN, Bedell V, Lipsey K, Macones GA, Cahill AG, Tuuli MG. Maternal marijuana use and adverse neonatal outcomes. *Obstetrics Gynecol.* 2016;128(4):713-723. doi:10.1097/aog.0000 000000001649.

[117] Metz T, Allshouse A. Maternal marijuana use, adverse pregnancy outcomes, and neonatal morbidity. *Am J Obstet Gynecol.* 2017;217(4):478.e1–8. doi:10.1016/j.ajog.2017.05.050.

[118] Leemaqz SY, Dekker GA, McCowan LM, et al. Maternal marijuana use has independent effects on risk for spontaneous preterm birth but not other common late pregnancy complications. *Reprod Toxicol.* 2016;62:77-86. doi:10.1016/j.reprotox.2016.04.021.

[119] Luke S, Hutcheon J, Kendall T. Cannabis use in pregnancy in British Columbia and selected birth outcomes. *J Obstetrics Gynaecol Can.* 2019;41. doi:10.1016/j.jogc.2018.11.014.

[120] Corsi D, Walsh L, Weiss D, Hsu H, El-Chaar D, Hawken S, Fell D, Walker M. Association between self-reported prenatal cannabis use and maternal, perinatal, and neonatal outcomes. JAMA 2019;322(2):145-152. doi.org: 10.1001/jama.2019.8734.

[121] Fried PA, James DS, Watkinson B. Growth and pubertal milestones during adolescence in offspring prenatally exposed to cigarettes and marihuana. *Neurotoxicol Teratol.* 2001;23(5):431-436. doi:10.1016/ s0892-0362(01)00161-1.

[122] Fried PA, Watkinson B, Gray R. Growth from birth to early adolescence in offspring prenatally exposed to cigarettes and marijuana. *Neurotoxicol Teratol.* 1999;21(5):513-525. doi:10.1016/ s0892-0362(99)00009-4.

[123] Kaul P, Bowker SL, Savu A, Yeung RO, Donovan LE, Ryan EA. Association between maternal diabetes, being large for gestational age and breast-feeding on being overweight or obese in childhood. *Diabetologia.* 2018;62(2):249-258. doi:10.1007/s00125-018-4758-0.

[124] Hamilton OJ, Fowose M, Colditz G, Tuuli MG, Carter EB. Cannabis use and fetal growth in pregnant women with diabetes [18L]. *Obstetrics Gynecol.* 2018;131:133S-134S. doi:10.1097/01.aog. 0000533557.76315.47.

[125] Halperin A. *Marijuana: Is it time to stop using a word with racist roots?* https://www.theguardian.com/society/2018/jan/29/marijuana-name-cannabis-racism. Published January 1, 2018. Accessed September 25, 2019.

[126] Shenassa ED, Kinsey C, Moser Jones M, Fahey J. Gestational Weight Gain: Historical evolution of a contested health outcome. *Obstet Gynecol Surv.* 2017;72(7):445-453. doi: 10.1097/OGX.00000 00000000459.

[127] Shenassa ED. Maternal smoking during pregnancy and offspring weight gain: A consideration of competing explanations. Paediatr Perinat Epidemiol. 2017 Sep;31(5):409-411. doi: 10.1111/ppe.12405.

In: New Research on Breastfeeding …
Editor: Kai Santos Melo

ISBN: 978-1-53617-061-0
© 2020 Nova Science Publishers, Inc.

Chapter 4

LESSONS FROM THE PAST: HOW RESEARCH, PROGRAMS AND LEGISLATION IMPACTED INFANT AND YOUNG CHILD NUTRITION FROM PREHISTORY TO THE END OF THE 19TH CENTURY

Veronika Scherbaum[1], PD, PhD
and Elizabeth Hormann[2]
[1]Institute for Biological Chemistry and Nutrition,
University of Hohenheim, Stuttgart, Germany
[2]European Institute for Breastfeeding and Lactation, Cologne, Germany

ABSTRACT

Recommendations and common feeding practices are closely linked with political and socio-economic conditions of different time periods and are embedded in culture-specific strategies for food, nutrition security and health care.

This narrative review addresses events and developments in the area of infant and young child nutrition as well as related research, programming and human rights issues from prehistory until the end of the 19th century. It also aims to draw key lessons from past findings and evolutions which took place in many societies and are highly relevant in today's context.

While artificial infant feeding has been always an important causal factor of child mortality, since middle of the 19th Century, environmental improvements and pasteurization of cow's milk have contributed to declining death rates. In addition, proper care and nutrition of young children with respect to health, growth and development as well as the essential role of a close mother-infant-relationship have been increasingly recognized. However, many socio-economic, cultural and legal constraints to support and protect adequate infant and young child feeding also play an important role.

INTRODUCTION

Efforts to safeguard infant and young child nutrition are part of the history of humankind. With the evolution of alimental concepts, growing knowledge, including trials and errors on nutritional needs of children, as well as legal protection and support, likely played an important role. But despite various efforts on different levels of societies, substantial numbers of children worldwide are not getting the nutrition they need to survive, grow and develop [1].

As the literature analysis has shown, over the course of 80 some years, many reviews of the history of young child nutrition have been published, from a general perspective [2-4], with a focus on specific sub-topics of child feeding [3, 5-11] or confined to distinct time periods or geographical contexts [9, 12-17].

The purpose of this narrative review is to address questions related to infant and young child nutrition from a historical perspective:

- Which relevant events, developments and important progress in research, programming and human rights took place in the past?
- What key lessons from past findings and dynamics, relevant for today's context can be drawn?

Apart from the difficulty in acknowledging the heterogeneity of societies with marked differences in food and nutritional conditions as well as socio-culturally determined feeding practices, reliable reports from Latin America, Asia and Africa on child health and nutrition up to the mid-20th century are rare. Thus, most available information was derived from industrialized countries.

Child Nutrition in Prehistoric Times

There is much evidence from early history about the importance of breastfeeding. This is shown in Mesolithic rock paintings and ancient sculptures of lactating women as well as the results of paleo-nutrition research, including the bone chemistry of skeletons more than 10,000 years old [6, 18, 19]. In addition to the intake of breastmilk, foods of animal origin as well as wild plants were offered, often after the time of dentition [4, 18, 20]. It is also assumed that pre-mastication of complementary foods by mothers played a crucial role in infant nutrition [21, 22].

Starting with the transition to agricultural societies, at around 10,000 years BC, and the ability to farm crops, cereals became the main constituents of complementary foods for infants [4, 6, 18, 20]. These foods consisted of semi-solid cereal 'paps', thin 'gruels' or 'panadas', or pulps, made of bread boiled in water or broth [23].

With the domestication of large mammals around 4,000 years BC, the introduction of animal milk and dairy products for young children began [24].

> **Specific Lessons Learned**
>
> Paleo-nutrition findings have underscored the role of breastfeeding in providing the "life fuel" for infants [19] within the close mother-infant relationship essential for child survival [25]. Despite incomplete and hypothetical knowledge about Paleolithic complementary foods [26], it is estimated that among pre-agricultural societies, the nutritional adequacy of these foods was higher and the prevalence of deficiencies in micronutrients, particularly iron and zinc, was lower than after the agricultural revolution [22]. Similarly, recent studies among contemporary groups of traditional hunters and gatherers revealed a higher diversity of the gut microbiota [27] than among rural farmers and even more compared with urban-industrialized populations [28]. This suggests a beneficial role for nutrient processing and absorption as well as immune protection [29] and the preservation of metabolic health [30].
>
> Cereal-based complementary foods, often given today as watery porridges [20] in many low-income countries, have a relatively low density and bioavailability of essential micronutrients [31]. As these deficiencies negatively affect child health, growth and development [22], current nutritional interventions aim to improve the diversity and composition of complementary foods and enhance the bioavailability of micronutrients [32-34].
>
> It has been suggested that the practice of pre-mastication of solid foods, which is still practiced by mothers in certain ethnic groups [35], is beneficial to the infant's digestion and absorption of micronutrients and may have additional immunological effects [21]. However, authors also critically point out that pre-mastication carries the risk of transmission of infectious pathogens such as hepatitis B, herpes simplex and HIV [36, 37].
>
> Currently, animal milk is seen in many societies as a "complete food" especially important for children [38, 39]. As a good source of high quality protein and micronutrients, such as calcium and vitamin B12 [40, 41], the addition of cow's milk to traditional cereal based diets of farmers has been considered beneficial for covering certain nutrient gaps [22, 42].
>
> The positive effects of milk-based complementary foods has been demonstrated by recent research [38, 43] documenting improved linear growth of young children [44]. However, the American Academy of Pediatrics in 1992 did not recommend the introduction of whole cow's milk for children under one year of age. [45]. Particular drawbacks were seen in the low content and bioavailability of iron, the high renal solute content, the risk of occult intestinal bleeding and its potential role as a food allergen [38, 46-48].

Young Child Feeding in Ancient Near East and Greco-Roman Civilizations

Among the ancient civilizations of Egypt and Mesopotamia, prolonged breastfeeding was widely practiced [3]. Similarly, in biblical Israel, children were seen as a gift from God. In the 2,000 year old Talmud, the particular quality of breastmilk was stressed, breastfeeding for two to four years was seen as a religious obligation "to preserve life", and social rights of breastfeeding mothers were emphasized [2, 3, 49]. In these civilizations, wet nursing was common. This became an organized profession with contracts and laws [11].

Specific Lessons Learned

There is sound evidence that continued breastfeeding for longer periods, as recommended in ancient civilizations, contributes to the health and well-being of both mothers and children [55-58]. According to international guidelines, children should be breastfed for up to two years or beyond, as mutually desired by both mother and child [59]. Compared with high income countries, the durations of breastfeeding are generally longer in low and middle income countries [60].

From early times, the practice of wet nursing was common in many societies until it eventually declined during the second half of the 19th century [3, 50]. During that time, the infant protection laws in France and England addressed the negative consequences of wet nursing on the nurse's own child and gave direction to later initiatives and legislation on maternal and child health in many countries [50].

Today, providing breastmilk of women other than the mother continues via certified milk banking for premature, low birthweight, sick and hospitalized newborns [61]. The provision of donor milk, which must meet specific quality standards [62, 63], is seen as a human rights issue [64] and is approved by WHO/UNICEF inclusive Infant and Young Child Feeding (IYCF) policies [65, 66].

Moreover, a growing demand for peer-to-peer breast milk sharing, e.g., via online communities in 50 countries, can be observed [67, 68]. This informal practice is not recommended by milk banking associations and La Leche League International due to known risks to safety and of adulteration, such as adding cow's milk [69-72]. Finally, in situations involving the absence, illness or death of mothers, such as during emergencies, 'cross nursing' of children by women other than the babies' own mothers [73] is still practiced in many cultures. In each of the concepts and practices mentioned, philosophical, cultural and religious motivations and objections must be taken into account [74, 75].

Effects of breastfeeding on psycho-emotional bonding between the mother and infant, involving positive maternal feelings and emotions towards the infant and long-term benefits for the child's cognitive and neurobehavioral development, are often mentioned in the literature [76-79]. It is plausible that social, sensory as well as endocrine factors, particularly the secretion of oxytocin and prolactin, contribute to fostering bonding [80, 81].

Among the attempts to assess the quality of breastmilk in antiquity, Soranus' fingernail test was of particular importance and was propagated for almost 2,000 years [82]. However, the marked differences between foremilk and hindmilk in appearance and composition, as well as color changes during the transition from the yellowish colostrum to mature human milk, which correspond to the newborn's specific needs, were not known in earlier times [83]. Research in recent decades on the belief that factors related to the mother or wet nurse may determine the quality of breast milk, has demonstrated some associations between maternal nutritional status and the mother's dietary intake and the nutrient content of breastmilk. These associations are in the amount and quality of fatty acids [84, 85] as well as certain water-soluble vitamins and trace elements, such as selenium and iodine [86-90]. In addition, maternal intake of substances; such as alcohol, nicotine, drugs and certain medications does have an impact on breastmilk [72].

The practice of withholding colostrum, often perceived as being dirty, and offering special prelacteal feeds to newborns instead [4] is found even today in many cultures worldwide [91-94].

Besides its nutritional properties, bioactive components of colostrum have been shown to enhance neonatal immune functions [95-98]. Its provision to the newborn is part of the WHO guidelines to promote early and exclusive breastfeeding, while the offering of any food or fluid other than breastmilk is discouraged [99].

In the Greco-Roman period, the role of breastfeeding in strengthening emotional bonds was increasingly recognized and the belief that character traits, including temperament and morals, were transmitted from wet nurses to the infant was widespread. Thus, the selection of a wet nurse according to qualification criteria grew in importance [3, 50-52].

Feeding a wet nurse's milk to newborns after delivery or offering pre-lacteal feeds, such as honey and butter, was recommended rather than giving colostrum, which was perceived as being impure [2, 4].

Besides human milk, animal milk, frequently given directly to young children from the udder of mammals, was propagated by Aristotle and the Greek physicians Galen and Soranus of Ephesus, who wrote the first texts on child care between 100 and 200 A.D. [4, 6]. According to Galen, excellent quality of mother's milk can be recognized by its pleasant taste and odor. It should be white, homogenous, and moderately thick [53]. Soranus described the "fingernail test" in his treatise to assess the consistency and quality of breastmilk [2, 54]:

> "If the droplet clings to the nail, it contains sufficient fat; if not, it is watery".

About 800 years later, another method for testing the quality and digestibility of breastmilk by adding rennet was introduced by the Byzantine physician Paulus Aegineta. His conclusions from the results of this test were [2]:

> "If the milk is too thick, the mother should be given emetics, to evacuate the phlegm, and if it is offensive, it should be expressed and the mother fed on fragrant food and wines".

Infant Feeding Recommendations until Post-Renaissance Time

The traditions of Greek, Byzantine and Arabic medicine were followed and expanded by the Persian physician and philosopher Avicenna (A.D.

980 to 1037) in the book 'Canon of Medicine'. Avicenna emphasized the need to ensure health, nutrition, hygiene and education from the earliest stages of life [100]. He also stressed the role of good health and nutrition of mothers during pregnancy and lactation.

Similar to Soranus, he advised mothers not to give colostrum to the newborn as it was thought to be harmful and not compatible with excreting meconium. Rather than colostrum, he recommended offering honey as a prelacteal food. However, he valued breastmilk as the most suitable food for infants and recommended that it should be given as long as possible. Avicenna's recommendations influenced newborn care and infant nutrition practices for some 600 years after his death [100-102].

During the Middle Ages, beliefs that physical and psychological characteristics are transmitted to a child via breastfeeding led to growing objections to wet nursing [11]. Children's deficits or illnesses were attributed to wet nurses' milk, compromised by diet, exercise, sexual activities and other lifestyle behaviors. While breastfeeding her own child was seen as a holy duty of a mother [51], offering animal milk to babies was discouraged because it was believed this would make the child 'animal-like' [3].

In the year 1513, 'Der Rosengarten', a book on infant feeding practices written by the German physician, Eucharius Roesslin, was published. By contrast to the most common practice of nursing infants for one year, he recommended breastfeeding for two years. Instead of sudden weaning, children should be slowly accustomed to family food by offering "little pills of bread" and sugar [2].

During the mid-16th century, the poem "Paedotrophia", written in Latin by the Frenchman Scevole de Ste. Marthe, was published and, over the next 200 years, was studied in European Universities [103]. On breastfeeding and weaning, it contained practical advice:

> ... "for suckling, no fix'd hour prescribe; This Nature teaches best the nursing tribe: Let her our mistress be; and when, with cries The hungry child demands his due supplies"...[103]

In his work 'The Nursing of Children' published in English in 1612, the French obstetrician, Jacques Guillemau, strongly exhorted women... "to nurse their own children themselves" and stressed that there "is no difference between a woman who refuses to nurse her own child, and one that kills her child as soon as she has conceived". Similarly, he was very critical of wet nursing and was convinced that the nurse's qualities conveyed via breastmilk were of greater importance than heredity by writing "nurture is more than nature" [104, 105].

Specific Lessons Learned

Avicenna highlighted the need for a life cycle perspective on health, nutrition and related areas. Over the last couple of decades, these concepts have become core elements of WHO/UNICEF strategies including 'Continuum of Care' across life stages [106, 107].

Avicenna has also stressed the benefits of breastfeeding and the essential importance of promoting the mother's well-being to ensure child health, growth and development.

Supported by the results of recent longitudinal studies, intervention packages for the different life stages, starting as early as pre-conception [108, 109], have been developed. These include the promotion of breastfeeding and adequate complementary feeding.

With respect to Roesslin's recommendation for a gradual process of weaning, this mode is seen as the most preferable if no medical or other mandatory reasons require abrupt weaning [110]. Generally, natural or baby-led weaning has to be distinguished from a planned or mother-led weaning approach [111]. The former advocates self-feeding of hand-held foods by the infant and the introduction of family foods, while spoon-feeding of puréed foods is omitted [112]. Studies have shown that the experiences of mothers with the feasibility of baby-led weaning and the adherence to this type of weaning vary greatly [113, 114]. There are still major unresolved issues on this type of weaning that require further investigation [115].

Ad-libitum breastfeeding propagated in the poem "Paedotrophia", is often seen as the most suitable practice involving the frequency and duration of lactation. Thus, feeding on demand is recommended as best practice and is included in the 10 Steps to Successful Breastfeeding guidance of the Baby Friendly Hospital Initiative [116], which itself is part of the IYCF-guidelines [117].

By contrast, 'scheduled breastfeeding' takes place when mothers feed their children on a predetermined and time restricted schedule [118]. This type of feeding, which became popular again during the 20th century [119], is viewed by critics as the result of increased medicalization of infant feeding [120]. Randomized controlled trials comparing the effects of the feeding modes do not exist and would be unlikely to receive ethical approval [118].

As mentioned in the book by the Countess of Lincoln, body image concerns have been a common objection to nursing a child. Even now, the fear that the firmness of breasts might be lost is known to influence the decision to breastfeed [121]. Studies have shown that risk factors for post-pregnancy breast ptosis increase with age, a higher body mass index, a greater number of pregnancies, a larger pre-pregnancy bra size, and smoking, while breastfeeding per se has been not found to be an independent risk factor for ptosis [122, 123].

In 1662, the book 'Countess of Lincoln Nurseries' was printed in Oxford on behalf of Elizabeth Clinton, dowager countess of Lincoln [50], who had given all of her 18 children to wet nurses and saw most of them die during infancy. When her daughter-in-law breastfed her own first child, which grew up healthy, she was ashamed and recognized her error. This motivated her to entreat other women to breastfeed.

> "...be not so unnatural to thrust away your own children".

Moreover, she rejected the-then current objections to breastfeeding, such as the opinion that nursing spoils the figure [105].

Pioneers in Promoting Young Child Health and Nutrition until the End of the 18th Century

While up to the beginning of the 18th century, half of all children in Europe died during the first year of life, the work of pediatricians drastically changed ideas that had persisted over many centuries. It was the German physician, Michael Ettmüller, (1644-83) in the book 'Ettmüller abridged', published by his son in 1702, who explicitly advised putting the child on the breast during the colostrum period. He also discouraged the use of pre-lacteal feeds in order to purge meconium, believed to be poisonous, and attempts to assess the quality of breastmilk by its thickness and taste [124]. .

The widely read pamphlet 'An Essay upon Nursing and the Management of Children from Their Birth to Three Years of Age' written in 1748 by the English physician William Cadogan who has been recognized as "the father of child care" had an enormous impact on child feeding practices [125].

Similar to Ettmüller, Cadogan propagated immediate attachment of the child to the mother's breast after delivery [125]:

> ... "it would suck with strength enough, after a few repeated trials, to make the milk flow gradually, in due proportion to the child's unexercised faculty of swallowing, and the call of its stomach"...

Specific Lessons Learned

While they condemned prelacteal feeds and recommended offering colostrum, both Ettmüller and Cadogan strongly propagated the *early initiation of breastfeeding*. And it was the special merit of Cadogan, who advised *skin-to-skin contact* and referred to sucking and let-down reflex patterns in the postnatal period [132].

According to WHO recommendations, the initiation of breastfeeding within 1 hour after birth is supported, when newborns are placed in skin-to-skin contact with their mothers immediately after birth [99]. It is suggested that uninterrupted intimate contact with self-attachment of the newborn to the mother's nipple is beneficial for effective nursing of the child and successful lactation [133]. Moreover, anxiety and stress levels of both the infant and the mother are thought to be lowered via complex neuro-endocrine regulation [134]. Similarly, the release of oxytocin seems to enhance maternal parenting confidence and contributes to improved mother-father-infant bonding [135]. Furthermore, positive long-term effects on the child, such as programming future physiology and psychosocial behavior, probably mediated through epigenetic changes [136], are postulated.

It has been shown that early initiation of breastfeeding is associated with reduced neonatal mortality [96, 137]. There is also evidence that it increases the likelihood of exclusive breastfeeding and the overall duration of breastfeeding [138]. Despite these positive impacts, the average prevalence in the world is still below 50% with wide differences between countries [139]. Major barriers are practices of prelacteal feeding and discarding colostrum, multiple births, complications during pregnancy, caesarean delivery and the lack of postnatal/neonatal care [140-142].

One of Cadogan's key messages is his recommendation to feed young infants exclusively with breastmilk. However, his statement on the duration of this feeding mode was rather vague and may have led to a delay in the introduction of complementary foods.

Promotion of e*xclusive breastfeeding* for six months, as recommended by WHO [143], is seen as one of the top priorities for reducing infant deaths [56]. It diminishes the risk of gastrointestinal infection, a major cause of under-five mortality in developing countries, and has beneficial effects on the mothers' health[144]. No deficits associated with the exclusiveness of feeding breastmilk were detected [145]. However, on average, only 40% of children younger than 6 months of age are exclusively breastfed worldwide [146].

In view of the high incidence of milk-borne infections as major causes of gastroenteritis, Cadogan's advice not to boil cow's milk has to be seen critically [147].

Similarly, Cadogan's recommendation to nurse infants with diarrhea only four times per day without feeding during the night might have had life-threatening consequences. Infants have to be breastfed frequently in order to prevent dehydration [148].

George Armstrong's dispensary for the infant poor provided curative services as well as counselling of mothers on child care, nutrition and hygiene. About 200 years later, comprehensive care became an integral part of the Primary Health Care (PHC) approach formulated in the Declaration of Alma Ata. This concept included promotion of food supplies and proper nutrition, safe water supplies and adequate sanitation as well as maternal and child health [149]. Similarly, curative and preventive components including counselling on proper young child nutrition constitute the concept of the Integrated Management of Childhood Illness (IMCI) applied today in Primary Health Care services in many countries worldwide [150].

George Armstrong's direct targeting of clinic health services to deprived families was particularly pioneering. With low-income settings today, the benefits of targeted health programs have been shown to reach the poorest households to a great extent [151]. This also applies for improvements in the knowledge of poor mothers and behavioral changes related to nutrition and hygiene through counselling and educational interventions [152].

Armstrong's advice to mothers tackles relevant topics of lactation and infant feeding, such as the prevention of mastitis with proper breastfeeding practices [153], maternal psycho-emotional influences on lactation [154] and the advantages of spoon feeding [155, 156] compared with bottle feeding by using perforated horns [11]. In addition, his recommendations on the time of introducing complementary foods and the transition to family foods are in accordance with current international guiding principles [157].

While condemning prelacteal feeds, he explicitly recommended feeding of colostrum and subsequent exclusive feeding of breastmilk for three to six months [125]

> ... "No child should ever be crammed with any unnatural mixture, till the provision of nature was ready for it; nor afterwards fed with any ungenial alien diet whatever"...

Cadogan recommended that cow's milk not be boiled because this alters the taste, destroys the sweetness and makes it "heavier" [124].

He also considered overfeeding to be a cause of diarrhea and advised women to breastfeed at regular intervals confined to four meals a day without any nursing during the night.

Cadogan was critical of the practice of wet nursing, commonly employed by wealthy women. On the other hand, he supported the employment of wet nurses to save lives of infants in foundling hospitals [125, 126].

In addition, he expressed the view that "men of sense rather than foolish unlearned women" have to be put in charge of infant care [95]. This view of men's role in supervising infant care was in line with the increasing scrutinization of midwifery and the management of infancy by medical men from the eighteenth century onwards [127].

The immense social inequalities in child morbidity and mortality were addressed by the physicians, John Armstrong and his younger brother George, in London. They opened the first clinic for children of poor families in 1769. George Armstrong identified inadequate knowledge of nutrition and hygiene among caregivers as an essential cause of early childhood illness and noted that the neglect of child health has the greatest consequences for the whole society [128, 129]. Apart from his curative work, Armstrong expended great effort on disease prevention

> ... "I always inquire into the diet of the children and give particular instruction about it, not only while they are ill, but also after they recovered" [129].

He recommended breastfeeding for the sake of the child and to prevent "milk fever" in the mother. Moreover, he wrote that anxious mothers sometimes make bad nurses. For children who had to be fed by hand, he advised using "new milk" offered by spoon, rather than by a horn [128]. At the age of 5 to 6 months, thickened feeds should be offered, gradually adding broth, beef tea, minced chicken and bread pudding [124].

Beginning in the second half of 17th century, the number of British upper- and middle class women who hired wet nurses, often organized by agencies, continuously increased [3]. For many poor women, wet nursing was a significant and continuous source of income at the expense of a diminished survival rate of their own children [50, 130]. As M.A. Baines expresses it in a Lancet article published later in 1867 [131]

> "Amongst its most disastrous results may be regarded the fate of the wet-nurse's child, which is in most cases put out to dry-nurse, falls into ignorant or unprincipled hands, and, as a consequence, too often meets with premature death"

The Development of Industrially Produced Breastmilk Substitutes

While over centuries, animal milk has been the most common source of artificial feeding, as early as 1610, Osswaldt Gaebelkhovern observed that infants fed with diluted cow's milk, enriched with cereal preparations, thrived better than those fed with undiluted milk [3]. Since the discovery by Johann Franz Simon in 1838 that cow's milk contains more protein and less carbohydrates than human milk [158, 159], dilution with water and subsequent addition of cereal preparations [3, 160] as well as sugar and cream [161] has been propagated.

In the middle of the 19th century, important technical inventions took place: in 1856 Gail Borden patented a vaporizer for the production of condensed milk; two years later, Ferdinand Carre developed the first water/ammonia absorption refrigerator and in 1860, the technique of pasteurization was discovered by Louis Pasteur [9].

> **Specific Lessons Learned**
>
> Gaebelkhovern's observation that breast milk substitutes prepared with diluted cow's milk and enriched with baked cereals are more wholesome than unmodified cow's milk is sound in view of the different nutrient content of cow's milk compared to human milk. The experience is that adding bread crumbs, biscuits or flour of baked or roasted cereals to infant foods is better tolerated by infants than fresh flour [23]. There is evidence that these processes improve the digestibility and bioavailability of the nutrients.
>
> Based on these experiences, 250 years later, industrially produced formulas were developed. Their use is indicated in situations in which breastmilk feeding cannot be achieved. However, quality standards must be safeguarded [170]. Home production of breastmilk substitutes should be avoided, as the nutrient composition, particularly the micronutrient content, usually differs significantly from breastmilk and cannot be adjusted at household level [171].
>
> Despite clear regulations since 1981 [172], marketing strategies of some companies continue to pretend that breastmilk substitutes are superior to human milk. Scientific evidence has disproved this [173]. Moreover, despite the conditions in low-income settings, negative consequences of using infant formula are often played down. These are life-threatening risks, such as severe gastroenteritis in infancy caused by contaminated water and undernutrition by over-dilution of formula. Furthermore, limited capabilities of caregivers to read and fully understand instructions on the label, may lead to under-dilution of formula with the risk of kidney damage due to high osmolality [174, 175].
>
> With condensed milk, which has been popular as an alternative to cow's milk in infant feeding [7], there have been reports from South East Asia in the last few decades, that certain brands have been promoted and used for decades as breastmilk substitutes with life-threatening consequences [176, 177].
>
> Since the determination of the macro- and micronutrient composition of human milk by Biedert and Meigs, an increasing variety of compounds, such as digestive enzymes, hormones, anti-inflammatory and anti-microbial factors, growth modulators and prebiotics have been detected [178, 179], while new breastmilk properties are still being identified. Despite immense efforts to "humanize" breastmilk substitutes, it is, as yet, impossible to produce formula with beneficial properties, which are anywhere near mothers' milk. This is due to the unique composition of human milk, which varies within feeds, diurnally and over lactation, dynamically adapting to the individual infant's needs [83].

In 1865, the German chemist, Justus von Liebig, invented a 'soup for nurslings' for his daughter's baby and eventually marketed the first industrially produced infant formula [161]. Compared to Liebig's product, which had to be mixed with preheated milk, the powdered 'Farine Lactée Nestlé', developed by Henry Nestlé in Switzerland in the year 1867, only needed to be mixed with boiled water. Through soaking zwieback in condensed milk, consecutive drying and grinding, a product was manufactured that could easily be sold in the countries of Europe and the USA [162].

While a growing demand for "clean alternatives" to breastmilk evolved, in 1879, the physician C.H.F. Routh, author of the book 'Infant feeding and its influence on Life' gave the first evidence that declining breastfeeding rates are a primary cause of infant mortality [163, 164].

In 1883, J.B. Meyenberg produced canned condensed milk with reduced sugar and adjusted fat content and, two years later, techniques of pasteurization were adopted for cow's milk by Franz von Soxhlet. He also discovered milk components, such as lactose and protein constituents, and the differences between these components in cow's and human milk [165]. In the same year, the nutrient composition of human milk and cow's milk was identified by Philipp Biedert in Germany and Charles Dulcena Meigs in the USA [166].

In later decades, the growing knowledge about the nutritional content of both types of milk stimulated attempts to "humanize" cow's milk, which led to extremely complicated methods of formula mixing [167-169].

Initiatives to Provide Pasteurized Milk and Social Justice Campaigns in the 19th Century

In England at the beginning of the 19th century, mothers engaged in paid work in urban factories far from their homes were forced to wean their infants early and feed them with cereal preparations or animal milk, usually under extremely poor hygienic conditions with a lack of clean water [3, 180]. Frequently, cow's milk was contaminated, as it had either been produced locally under dirty conditions or transported long distances to the cities. In addition, the milk was adulterated by diluting it with water or by adding substances, such as chalk and flour [147]. Under these circumstances, artificial feeding of infants commonly resulted in diarrheal diseases and a high prevalence of malnutrition, which contributed to extremely high rates of infant mortality [181, 182]. A specific tragic fate was observed among many children of wet nurses. In addition to the consequences of dry nursing, some of these children experienced poor care or even infanticide in "baby farms". This eventually led to the 'Infant Life Protection Act' in England in the year 1870 and the law 'for the protection of infants sent out to nurse' in France 1874 [50].

In the second half of the 19th century, environmental improvements, mandatory milk pasteurization laws, "clean milk movements", "save the babies" campaigns and the provision of sterilized and pasteurized milk played an increasing role in infant welfare programs in European countries and the USA [147, 183]. These initiatives contributed to a marked decline in infant mortality [184-187].

In the 1890s, pasteurized cow's milk began to be provided in some consultation services and dispensaries in France to mothers who were unable to breastfeed. The first services of this kind were set up by Pierre Constant Budin who opened a perinatal consultation service in the Charité hospital in Paris 1892 and by Leon Dufour in Normandy in 1894. Simultaneously, both men propagated the importance of exclusive breastfeeding. As a co-founder of the "League against infant mortality", Budin was concerned with the high death rates in early childhood, while other contemporary pediatricians usually focused on the health of children older than two [188]. He monitored the nutritional status of young infants with special growth charts and observed a significant reduction in infant mortality rates when mothers received counselling in proper nutrition and prevention of infectious diseases [189, 190]. Moreover, he outlined principles for care of the "weaklings", as premature, sick and low birth weight infants were called, with particular emphasis on warmth, cleanliness and early breastfeeding. He was influenced in his approaches in perinatology by his predecessor and teacher at the maternal hospital in Paris, Stéphane Tarnier, considered the dean of obstetrics to whom, *inter alia*, the use of incubator care and "gavage feeding" of preterm infants by gastric tube is attributed [191, 192]. Budin who carried on Tarnier's work, gave these instructions on the nutrition of the preterm baby:

..."if the child does not wish to take the breast, or is not strong enough to suck, it must be fed from a spoon, and if it cannot swallow, gavage must be employed" [189].

Furthermore, Budin established procedures to enhance mother-infant bonding: He introduced glass incubators, allowing mothers to see their babies at the bedside, and recommended a rapid switch from the breastmilk of wet nurses, as far as initially needed, to mother's own milk as soon as it appeared [193]. In his textbook "Le Nourrisson" (The Nursling) [192], published later, Budin stressed the importance of treating premature infants born at the hospital and emphasized that the mother's presence and early involvement in the care and proper feeding of vulnerable infants are essential for their survival after discharge

... "save the infant in such a way that when it leaves the hospital it does it with a mother able to suckle it" [192].

It must be noted however, that Budin's efforts for the survival of most vulnerable babies were rejected by proponents of *eugenics* movements, who argued that these individuals, whose lives had been saved, remain infirm for a lifetime [193, 194].

Besides the initiatives in France focusing on the critical neonatal period [195], health and nutrition aspects of young children were addressed by infant welfare centers, first established in England in 1890, which provided home visits with counselling in infant health and the nutrition of caregivers [195].

While in the 19th century, the vast majority of infants were nourished at their mothers' breasts, the pediatric theory that maternal breastmilk represents the only safe and healthful infant food began to change towards the end of that century [196, 197]. As clearly seen in the USA, cultural change associated with ongoing urbanization and rapid industrialization, including the adoption of feeding schedules with long intervals, took place. This led a growing number of women from all classes to start artificial feeding or mixed feeding from birth onwards or to wean in the third month or even before. During this time, perceptions of mothers having "lactation failure" became more and more widespread. As a consequence, several pediatricians began to question the adequacy of breastmilk in terms of quantity and quality.

Specific Lessons Learned

The fact that economic needs forced mothers of the urban labor class as well as wet nurses to wean their children at a very young age was a great tragedy. Even now, in low-income settings, artificially fed infants, by comparison to those exclusively breastfed, have a risk of dying from diarrhea that is approximately 10 times higher and they are 15 times more likely to die from pneumonia [201]. Thus, measures to ensure parental leave and breastfeeding support at the workplace have the potential to improve child health outcomes worldwide [202, 203].

The clean milk movement and the mandatory pasteurization of milk, as well as the opening of milk depots, led to a reduction of infant deaths caused by milk-borne diseases in Europe and the USA. However, these developments also contributed to an increased use of cow's milk as a breastmilk substitute and, consequently, led to a decline in breastfeeding rates. This, in turn, fostered the process of industrial production of breastmilk substitutes and their marketing worldwide [204].

Budin, along with Tarnier, can be seen as the fathers of modern perinatal/neonatal medicine, whose pioneering work in the care of premature infants is still of greatest relevance today. Apart from the fact that prematurity and its complications are the main causes of under-5 mortality [205], the increased risk of preterm infants developing certain non-communicable diseases in later life and the burden of prematurity-related disability are still major public health concerns [206].

The inclusion of mothers in hospital care aiming to achieve active mother-infant bonding, as Budin emphasized, are an important component of today's family integrated care concepts offering parents access to their babies in neonatal care units. It has been demonstrated that this model leads to improved infant weight gain, decreased parent stress and anxiety as well as the high-frequency of exclusive breastfeeding at discharge [207], while positive effects of maternal breastfeeding by increasing self-efficacy are suggested [208]. Similarly, gavage feeding promoted by Tarnier and Budin for vulnerable babies not able to effectively feed at the breast, by bottle or spoon for medical or physiological reasons, is still practiced in neonatal and maternity units [209]. Study results suggest that simultaneous non-nutritive sucking on a pacifier encourages the development of sucking behavior and improves the transition from gavage to full oral feeding [210].

The efforts of Tarnier and Budin to prevent hypothermia in preterm and low birthweight babies with the use of incubators are also part of today's intensive thermal care of vulnerable infants. The same applies for Kangaroo Mother Care, which significantly contributes to improved health outcomes in these babies [211, 212]. This simple method provides stable warmth through early and continuous skin-to-skin contact between the baby and the mother and facilitates frequent and exclusive provision of mother's breastmilk [209] which was considered a key principle of care even more than 100 years ago.

Mothers' perceptions of not producing breastmilk of sufficient quantity and quality are still widespread today. Consequently, this leads to early weaning and increased use of formula [213]. Apart from the fact that many mothers do not know that the amount of breastmilk depends on the frequency of sucking at the breast, the perceived insufficient milk (PIM) dilemma is often fostered by other persons' views.

The social justice movements in the late 19th century already emphasized proper child care and nutrition, including breastfeeding as a right of both the mother and the child. [214]. Today, these rights are fixed in the broader context of the human right to adequate food and the Convention on the Rights of the Child in international human rights law and principles. As adequate national policies and legislation in many societies are lacking, the demands are still relevant today.

At the end of the 19th century, it became also clear that pathogens, such as bacteria, were eventually found to be the causes of gastroenteritis accounting for the high infant mortality. While many healthcare workers endeavored to mitigate the disastrous effects of unsanitary artificial feeding, instead of promoting breastfeeding, pediatricians emphasized the need to improve artificial feeding, including the demand for high quality breast milk substitutes as public health priorities [198, 199].

As a counterpoint, health reformers and activists articulated that a child's right for equal access to human milk as well as a mother's ability to adequately care for her babies are fundamental aspects of social justice [187, 198]. At the end of the 19th century, grassroots organizations, formed by mothers in countries, such as Germany, Britain and France, demanded that their governments support mothers to better care for their babies. This was the beginning of many crusades of social activism for infant and maternal health continuing until World War I [200].

CONCLUSION

This review of historical events and developments in young child feeding has been an attempt to illustrate the evolution of today's strategies aiming to improve the social, nutritional and health conditions of young children, who are the most vulnerable in any society.

Even in the 19th century, childhood was increasingly understood as a time which needs specific protection and support. Moreover, the essential role of a close mother-infant-relationship, as well as proper care and nutrition, in the health, growth and development of the individual had been recognized. Similarly, attitudes on wet nursing changed continuously. At the same time, a growing demystification of taboos inhibiting early initiation of exclusive breastfeeding was noticeable. For many centuries, artificial infant feeding was an important causal factor of child mortality, while improvements in hygiene and the invention of pasteurization for cow's milk contributed to declining death rates. Despite these developments, the need to promote, support and protect breastfeeding as an optimal mode of infant and young child feeding has remained relevant until today.

REFERENCES

[1] UNICEF. *Adopting optimal feeding practices is fundamental to a child's survival, growth and development, but too few children benefit* - See more at: http://data.unicef.org/nutrition/iycf#sthash. uMDBNMxR.dpuf. New York: UNICEF; 2015.

[2] Wickes IG. A history of infant feeding. I. Primitive peoples; ancient works; Renaissance writers. *Arch Dis Child.* 1953 Apr;28(138):151-8.

[3] Fildes VA. Breasts, Bottles and Babies: A history of infant feeding. *Edinburgh: Edinburgh Univ Pr;* 1986.

[4] Castilho SD and Barros Filho AA. The history of infant nutrition. *J Pediatr (Rio J).* 2010 May-Jun;86(3):179-88.

[5] Lyon AB. History of Infant Feeding. *Am J Dis Child.* 1933;46(2):359-74.

[6] Tönz O. Stillpraxis im Wandel der Zeit (Breastfeeding practice through the ages). In: Scherbaum V, Perl FM and Kretschmer U (eds). *Stillen, Frühkindliche Ernährung und reproduktive Gesundheit* [*Breastfeeding, Early Childhood Nutrition and Reproductive Health*] Köln: Deutscher Ärzte-Verlag; 2003. p. 1-6.

[7] Bryder L. From breast to bottle: a history of modern infant feeding. *Endeavour.* 2009 Jun; 33(2):54-9.

[8] Droese W. Zur Geschichte der Beikost in der Säuglingsernährung [On the history of complementary foods in infant nutrition]. In: Ewerbeck H (ed). *Beikost in der Säuglingsernährung* [*Complementary Foods in Infant Nutrition*]. Berlin: Springer; 1985. p. 111-7.

[9] Obladen M. Technical inventions that enabled artificial infant feeding. *Neonatology.* 2014;106(1):62-8.

[10] Papageorgopoulou C, Staub K and Rühli F. *Hypothyroidism in Switzerland*. Sickness, Hunger, War, and Religion München: RCC 2012. p. 75-90.

[11] Stevens EE, Patrick TE and Pickler R. A History of Infant Feeding. *J Perinat Educ.* 2009 Spring;18(2):32-9.

[12] Weaver LT. How did babies grow 100 years ago? *Eur J Clin Nutr.* 2011 Jan;65(1):3-9.

[13] Weaver LT. The emergence of our modern understanding of infant nutrition and feeding 1750-1900 *Current Paediatrics* 2006;16:342-7.

[14] Fomon S. Infant feeding in the 20th century: formula and beikost. *J Nutr.* 2001 Feb;131(2):409S-20S.

[15] Anderson S. Then and now: infant feeding in Britain, 1900-1914. *Prof Care Mother Child.* 1996;6(6):167, 70.

[16] Forsyth D. The History of Infant-feeding from Elizabethan Times. *Proc R Soc Med.* 1911;4(Sect Study Dis Child):110-41.

[17] Fulminante F. Infant Feeding Practices in Europe and the Mediterranean from Prehistory to the Middle Ages: A Comparison between the Historical Sources and Bioarchaeology. *Childhood in the Past: An International Journal.* 2015;8(1):24-47.

[18] Dettwyler KA. Breastfeeding in Prehistory. In: Stuart-MacAdam P and Dettwyler KA (eds). *Breastfeeding Biocultural Perspectives.* Chicago: Aldine Transaction; 1995. p. 76-102.

[19] Uva BA. *Breasts are for Feeding: An Anthropological, Archaeological Examination of Breastfeeding* San Luis Obispo: California Polytechnic State University; 2011.

[20] Larsen CS. Animal source foods and human health during evolution. *J Nutr.* 2003 Nov;133(11 Suppl 2):3893S-7S.

[21] Pelto GH, Zhang Y and Habicht JP. Premastication: the second arm of infant and young child feeding for health and survival? *Matern Child Nutr.* 2011 Jan;6(1):4-18.

[22] Dewey KG. The challenge of meeting nutrient needs of infants and young children during the period of complementary feeding: an evolutionary perspective. *J Nutr.* 2013 Dec;143(12):2050-4.

[23] Obladen M. Pap, gruel, and panada: early approaches to artificial infant feeding. *Neonatology.* 2014;105(4):267-74.

[24] Lacaille AD. Infant feeding-bottles in prehistoric times. *Proc R Soc Med.* 1950 Jul;43(7):565-8.

[25] Stuart-Macadam P. Breastfeeding in Prehistory. In: Stuart-Macadam P and Dettwyler KA (eds). *Breastfeeding Biocultural Perspectives.* Chicago: Transaction Publishers; 1995. p. 76-102.

[26] Nestle M. Paleolithic diets: a sceptical view. *Nutrition Bulletin.* 2000;25(1):43-7.

[27] Obregon-Tito AJ, Tito RY, Metcalf J, Sankaranarayanan K, Clemente JC, Ursell LK, Zech Xu Z, Van Treuren W, Knight R, Gaffney PM, Spicer P, Lawson P, Marin-Reyes L, Trujillo-Villarroel O, Foster M, Guija-Poma E, Troncoso-Corzo L, Warinner C, Ozga AT and Lewis CM. Subsistence strategies in traditional societies distinguish gut microbiomes. *Nat Commun.* 2015 Mar 25;6:6505.

[28] Gupta VK, Paul S and Dutta C. Geography, Ethnicity or Subsistence-Specific Variations in Human Microbiome Composition and Diversity. *Front Microbiol.* 2017;8:1162.

[29] Kau AL, Ahern PP, Griffin NW, Goodman AL and Gordon JI. Human nutrition, the gut microbiome and the immune system. *Nature.* 2011 Jun 15; 474 (7351):327-36.

[30] Joyce SA and Gahan CG. The gut microbiota and the metabolic health of the host. *Curr Opin Gastroenterol.* 2014 Mar;30(2):120-7.

[31] Dewey KG and Brown KH. Update on technical issues concerning complementary feeding of young children in developing countries and implications for intervention programs. *Food Nutr Bull.* 2003 Mar;24(1):5-28.

[32] Hotz C and Gibson RS. Traditional food-processing and preparation practices to enhance the bioavailability of micronutrients in plant-based diets. *J Nutr.* 2007 Apr;137(4):1097-100.

[33] Waswa LM, Jordan I, Herrmann J, Krawinkel MB and Keding GB. Community-based educational intervention improved the diversity

of complementary diets in western Kenya: results from a randomized controlled trial. *Public Health Nutr.* 2015 Apr 10:1-14.

[34] FAO. *Participatory nutrition education catalyst for dietary diversity.* Lilongwe, Malawi: FAO Regional Office for Africa; 2015.

[35] Jellife DB. *Infant nutrition in the Subtropics and Tropics, WHO Monograph Series.* Geneva: WHO; 1968.

[36] Dinubile MJ. Premastication: a possible missing link? *Clin Infect Dis.* 2010 Jul 15;51(2):252-3.

[37] Levison J, Gillespie SL and Montgomery E. Think twice before recommending pre-masticated food as a source of infant nutrition. *Matern Child Nutr.* 2011 Jan;7(1):104; author reply 5-6.

[38] Allen LH and Dror DK. Effects of animal source foods, with emphasis on milk, in the diet of children in low-income countries. *Nestle Nutr Workshop Ser Pediatr Program.* 2011;67:113-30.

[39] Scherbaum V and Srour ML. Milk products in the dietary management of childhood undernutrition - a historical review. *Nutr Res Rev.* 2018 Jun;31(1):71-84.

[40] Michaelsen KF. Cows' milk in complementary feeding. *Pediatrics.* 2000 Nov;106(5):1302-3.

[41] Pereira PC. Milk nutritional composition and its role in human health. *Nutrition.* 2014 Jun;30(6):619-27.

[42] Sadler K, Kerven C, Calo M and Catley A. *Milk Matters: A literature review of pastoralist nutrition and programming responses.* Addis Ababa; 2009.

[43] Molgaard C, Larnkjaer A, Arnberg K and Michaelsen KF. Milk and growth in children: effects of whey and casein. *Nestle Nutr Workshop Ser Pediatr Program.* 2011;67:67-78.

[44] Yackobovitch-Gavan M, Phillip M and Gat-Yablonski G. How Milk and Its Proteins Affect Growth, Bone Health, and Weight. *Horm Res Paediatr.* 2017 Mar 02.

[45] AAP. *The Use of Whole Cow's Milk in Infancy:* American Academy on Pediatrics, Committee on Nutrition. Pediatrics; 1992.

[46] Ziegler EE. Consumption of cow's milk as a cause of iron deficiency in infants and toddlers. *Nutr Rev.* 2011 Nov;69 Suppl 1:S37-42.

[47] Domellof M, Braegger C, Campoy C, Colomb V, Decsi T, Fewtrell M, Hojsak I, Mihatsch W, Molgaard C, Shamir R, Turck D and van Goudoever J. Iron requirements of infants and toddlers. *J Pediatr Gastroenterol Nutr.* 2014 Jan;58(1):119-29.

[48] Ziegler EE. Adverse effects of cow's milk in infants. *Nestle Nutr Workshop Ser Pediatr Program.* 2007;60:185-96; discussion 96-9.

[49] Eidelman AI. The Talmud and human lactation: the cultural basis for increased frequency and duration of breastfeeding among Orthodox Jewish women. *Breastfeed Med.* 2006 Spring;1(1):36-40.

[50] Obladen M. Regulated wet nursing: managed care or organized crime? *Neonatology.* 2012;102(3):222-8.

[51] Osborn ML. The rent breasts. Part II. *Midwife Health Visit Community Nurse.* 1979 Sep;15(9):347-8.

[52] Thorley V and Sioda T. Selection criteria for wet-nurses: Ancient recommendations that survived across time. *Breastfeed Rev.* 2016 Nov;24(3):13-24.

[53] Papastavrou M, Genitsaridi SM, Komodiki E, Paliatsou S, Kontogeorgou A and Iacovidou N. Breastfeeding in the Course of History. *Journal of Pediatrics and Neonatal Care* 2015;2(6).

[54] Luecke PE, Jr. *The history of pediatrics at Baylor University Medical Center.* Proc (Bayl Univ Med Cent). 2004 Jan;17(1):56-60.

[55] Chowdhury R, Sinha B, Sankar MJ, Taneja S, Bhandari N, Rollins N, Bahl R and Martines J. Breastfeeding and maternal health outcomes: a systematic review and meta-analysis. *Acta Paediatr.* 2015 Dec;104(467):96-113.

[56] Victora CG, Bahl R, Barros AJ, Franca GV, Horton S, Krasevec J, Murch S, Sankar MJ, Walker N and Rollins NC. Breastfeeding in the 21st century: Epidemiology, mechanisms, and lifelong effect. *Lancet.* 2016 Jan 30;387(10017):475-90.

[57] Horta BL, Loret de Mola C and Victora CG. Long-term consequences of breastfeeding on cholesterol, obesity, systolic blood

pressure and type 2 diabetes: A systematic review and meta-analysis. *Acta Paediatr.* 2015 Dec;104(467):30-7.

[58] Horta BL, Loret de Mola C and Victora CG. Breastfeeding and intelligence: A systematic review and meta-analysis. *Acta Paediatr.* 2015 Dec;104(467):14-9.

[59] WHO. *Continued breastfeeding for healthy growth and development of children.* e-Library of Evidence for Nutrition Actions (eLENA) 2018 [cited; Available from: http://www.who.int/elena/titles/continued_breastfeeding/en/

[60] UNICEF. *Breastfeeding. A Mother's Gift, for Every Child* New York: UNICEF; 2018.

[61] Kim J and Unger S. Human milk banking. *Paediatr Child Health.* 2010 Nov;15(9):595-602.

[62] Springer S. Umgang mit Muttermilch bei Trennung von Mutter und Kind. (Handling mother's milk when mother and child are separated) In: Scherbaum V, Perl FM and Kretschmer U (eds.). *Stillen, Frühkindliche Ernährung und reproduktive Gesundheit. (Breastfeeding, Early Childhood Nutrition and Reproductive Health)* Köln: Deutscher Ärzteverlag 2003. p. 152-8.

[63] Landers S and Hartmann BT. Donor human milk banking and the emergence of milk sharing. *Pediatr Clin North Am.* 2013 Feb;60(1):247-60.

[64] Arnold LD. Global health policies that support the use of banked donor human milk: A human rights issue. *Int Breastfeed J.* 2006;1:26.

[65] WHO/UNICEF. WHO/UNICEF meeting on infant and young child feeding. *J Nurse Midwifery.* 1980 May-Jun;25(3):31-9.

[66] WHO/UNICEF. *Global Strategy for Infant and Young Child Feeding.* Geneva: WHO; 2003.

[67] Martino K and Spatz D. Informal milk sharing: What nurses need to know. *MCN Am J Matern Child Nurs.* 2014 Nov-Dec;39(6):369-74.

[68] Akre JE, Gribble KD and Minchin M. Milk sharing: From private practice to public pursuit. *Int Breastfeed J.* 2011;6:8.

[69] Keim SA, McNamara KA, Jayadeva CM, Braun AC, Dillon CE and Geraghty SR. Breast milk sharing via the internet: The practice and health and safety considerations. *Matern Child Health J.* 2014 Aug;18(6):1471-9.

[70] Gribble KD and Hausman BL. Milk sharing and formula feeding: Infant feeding risks in comparative perspective? *Australas Med J.* 2012;5(5):275-83.

[71] St-Onge M, Chaudhry S and Koren G. Donated breast milk stored in banks versus breast milk purchased online. *Can Fam Physician.* 2015 Feb;61(2):143-6.

[72] Baumgartel KL, Sneeringer L and Cohen SM. From royal wet nurses to Facebook: The evolution of breastmilk sharing. *Breastfeed Rev.* 2016 Nov;24(3):25-32.

[73] Krantz JZ and Kupper NS. Cross-nursing: Wet-nursing in a contemporary context. *Pediatrics.* 1981 May;67(5):715-7.

[74] Ozdemir R, Ak M, Karatas M, Ozer A, Dogan DG and Karadag A. Human milk banking and milk kinship: Perspectives of religious officers in a Muslim country. *J Perinatol.* 2015 Feb;35(2):137-41.

[75] Gribble KD. Peer-to-peer milk donors' and recipients' experiences and perceptions of donor milk banks. *J Obstet Gynecol Neonatal Nurs.* 2013 Jul;42(4):451-61.

[76] Leung AK and Sauve RS. Breast is best for babies. *J Natl Med Assoc.* 2005 Jul;97(7):1010-9.

[77] Dieterich CM, Felice JP, O'Sullivan E and Rasmussen KM. Breastfeeding and health outcomes for the mother-infant dyad. Pediatr Clin North Am. 2013 Feb;60(1):31-48.

[78] Liu J, Leung P and Yang A. Breastfeeding and active bonding protects against children's internalizing behavior problems. *Nutrients.* 2013 Jan;6(1):76-89.

[79] Kramer MS, Aboud F, Mironova E, Vanilovich I, Platt RW, Matush L, Igumnov S, Fombonne E, Bogdanovich N, Ducruet T, Collet JP, Chalmers B, Hodnett E, Davidovsky S, Skugarevsky O, Trofimovich O, Kozlova L and Shapiro S. Breastfeeding and child

cognitive development: New evidence from a large randomized trial. *Arch Gen Psychiatry.* 2008 May;65(5):578-84.

[80] Kendrick KM. Oxytocin, motherhood and bonding. *Exp Physiol.* 2000 Mar;85 Spec No:111S-24S.

[81] Jansen J, de Weerth C and Riksen-Walraven JM. Breastfeeding and the mother–infant relationship—A review. *Developmental Review.* 2008;28(4):503-21.

[82] AAP. Soranus (A.D. 98-138) of Ephesus'Fingernail Method of testing the Quality of Breast Milk - a Clinical Test widely used for almost 20 Centuries. *Pediatrics.* 1969;44(6):972.

[83] Riordan JM. The biological specifity of breast milk In: Riordan JM and Wambach K (eds). *Breastfeeding and human lactation.* Burlington MA: Jones and Bartlett Learning 2010. p. 117-51.

[84] Anderson AK, McDougald DM and Steiner-Asiedu M. Dietary trans fatty acid intake and maternal and infant adiposity. *Eur J Clin Nutr.* 2010 Nov;64(11):1308-15.

[85] Kim J and Friel J. Lipids and Human Milk. *Lipid Technology.* 2012;24(5):103-5.

[86] Gushurst CA, Mueller JA, Green JA and Sedor F. Breast milk iodide: Reassessment in the 1980s. *Pediatrics.* 1984 Mar;73(3):354-7.

[87] Mannan S and Picciano MF. Influence of maternal selenium status on human milk selenium concentration and glutathione peroxidase activity. *Am J Clin Nutr.* 1987 Jul;46(1):95-100.

[88] Kang-Yoon SA, Kirksey A, Giacoia G and West K. Vitamin B-6 status of breast-fed neonates: Influence of pyridoxine supplementation on mothers and neonates. *Am J Clin Nutr.* 1992 Sep;56(3):548-58.

[89] Brannon PM and Picciano MF. Vitamin D in pregnancy and lactation in humans. *Annu Rev Nutr.* 2012 Aug 21;31:89-115.

[90] Picciano MF. Pregnancy and lactation: Physiological adjustments, nutritional requirements and the role of dietary supplements. *J Nutr.* 2003 Jun;133(6):1997S-2002S.

[91] Getahun Z, Scherbaum V, Taffese Y, Teshome B and Biesalski HK. Breastfeeding in Tigray and Gonder, Ethiopia, with special reference to exclusive/almost exclusive breastfeeding beyond six months. *Breastfeed Rev.* 2004 Nov;12(3):8-16.

[92] Morse JM, Jehle C and Gamble D. Initiating breastfeeding: A world survey of the timing of postpartum breastfeeding. *Int J Nurs Stud.* 1990;27(3):303-13.

[93] Inayati DA, Scherbaum V, Purwestri RC, Hormann E, Wirawan NN, Suryantan J, Hartono S, Bloem MA, Pangaribuan RV, Biesalski HK, Hoffmann V and Bellows AC. Infant feeding practices among mildly wasted children: A retrospective study on Nias Island, Indonesia. *Int Breastfeed J.* 2012;7(1):3.

[94] Ahmed FU, Rahman ME and Alam MS. Prelacteal feeding: Influencing factors and relation to establishment of lactation. *Bangladesh Med Res Counc Bull.* 1996 Aug;22(2):60-4.

[95] Wambach K and Riordan JM (eds). *Breastfeeding and Human Lactation*. 5 ed. Burlington: Jones and Bartlett; 2014.

[96] Edmond KM, Zandoh C, Quigley MA, Amenga-Etego S, Owusu-Agyei S and Kirkwood BR. Delayed breastfeeding initiation increases risk of neonatal mortality. *Pediatrics.* 2006 Mar;117(3):e380-6.

[97] Debes AK, Kohli A, Walker N, Edmond K and Mullany LC. Time to initiation of breastfeeding and neonatal mortality and morbidity: A systematic review. *BMC Public Health.* 2013;13 Suppl 3:S19.

[98] Khan J, Vesel L, Bahl R and Martines JC. Timing of Breastfeeding Initiation and Exclusivity of Breastfeeding During the First Month of Life: Effects on Neonatal Mortality and Morbidity-A Systematic Review and Meta-analysis. *Matern Child Health J.* 2014 Mar;19(3):468-79.

[99] WHO. *Early initiation of breastfeeding to promote exclusive breastfeedin.* e-Library of Evidence for Nutrition Actions (eLENA) 2018 [cited; Available from: http://www.who.int/elena/titles/early_breastfeeding/en/

[100] Borhani Nejad M, Rashidi M and Oloumi MM. Avicenna's Educational Views with Emphasis on the Education of Hygiene and Wellness. *Int J Health Policy Manag.* 2013 Sep;1(3):201-5.

[101] Modanlou HD. Avicenna (AD 980 to 1037) and the care of the newborn infant and breastfeeding. *J Perinatol.* 2008 Jan;28(1):3-6.

[102] Dunn PM. Avicenna (AD 980-1037) and Arabic perinatal medicine. *Arch Dis Child Fetal Neonatal Ed.* 1997 Jul;77(1):F75-6.

[103] Dunn PM. Scevole de Ste Marthe of France (1536-1623) and The Paedotrophia. *Arch Dis Child.* 1992 Apr;67(4 Spec No):468-9.

[104] Guillemau J. *The nursing of a child.* San Francisco: University of California. Medical Center library. Online collection Publication from 1612.

[105] Wickes IG. A history of infant feeding. II. Seventeenth and eighteenth centuries. *Arch Dis Child.* 1953 Jun;28(139):232-40; contd.

[106] PMNCH. Reaching Every Woman and Every Child through Partnership. *Working together to improve the health of women and children.* Geneva; 2013.

[107] Kerber KJ, de Graft-Johnson JE, Bhutta ZA, Okong P, Starrs A and Lawn JE. Continuum of care for maternal, newborn, and child health: From slogan to service delivery. *Lancet.* 2007 Oct 13;370(9595):1358-69.

[108] WHO. *Meeting to Develop a Global Consensus on Preconception Care to Reduce Maternal and Childhood Mortality and Morbidity.* Geneva: WHO; 2012.

[109] Brown JE. Preconception Nutrition. In: Brown JE, Isaaks J, Krinke B, *Lechtenberg E and Murtaugh M* (eds). Nutrition Through the Life Cycle: Wadsworth-Cengage; 2013. p. 50-70.

[110] N.A. Weaning your child from breastfeeding. *Paediatr Child Health.* 2004 Apr;9(4):254-65.

[111] N.A. Weaning from the breast. *Paediatr Child Health.* 2004 Apr;9(4):249-63.

[112] Brown A and Lee M. A descriptive study investigating the use and nature of baby-led weaning in a UK sample of mothers. *Matern Child Nutr.* 2011 Jan;7(1):34-47.

[113] D'Andrea EMR, Jenkins KMRC, Mathews MP and Roebothan BRP. Baby-led Weaning: A Preliminary Investigation. *Can J Diet Pract Res.* 2016 Jan 15:1-6.

[114] Cameron SL, Heath AL and Taylor RW. How feasible is Baby-led Weaning as an approach to infant feeding? A review of the evidence. N*utrients.* 2012 Nov;4(11):1575-609.

[115] D'Auria E, Bergamini M, Staiano A, Banderali G, Pendezza E, Penagini F, Zuccotti GV and Peroni DG. Baby-led weaning: What a systematic review of the literature adds on. *Ital J Pediatr.* 2018 May 3;44(1):49.

[116] WHO and UNICEF. *Baby Friendly Hospital Initiative Revised, Updated and Expanded for Integrated Care .* Geneva; 2009.

[117] UNICEF. *Programming Guide: Infant and Young Child Feeding.* New York: UNICEF; 2011.

[118] Fallon A, Van der Putten D, Dring C, Moylett EH, Fealy G and Devane D. Baby-led compared with scheduled (or mixed) breastfeeding for successful breastfeeding. *Cochrane Database Syst Rev.* 2014;7:CD009067.

[119] Manz F, van't Hof MA and Haschke F. The mother-infant relationship: Who controls breastfeeding frequency? Euro-Growth Study Group. *Lancet.* 1999 Apr 3;353(9159):1152.

[120] Palmer G (ed). *The Politics of Breastfeeding: When Breasts are Bad for Business.* 3 ed. London: Pinter & Martin; 2009.

[121] Brown A, Rance J and Warren L. Body image concerns during pregnancy are associated with a shorter breast feeding duration. *Midwifery.* 2015 Jan;31(1):80-9.

[122] Rinker B, Veneracion M and Walsh CP. The effect of breastfeeding on breast aesthetics. *Aesthet Surg J.* 2008 Sep-Oct;28(5):534-7.

[123] Pisacane A and Continisio P. Breastfeeding and perceived changes in the appearance of the breasts: A retrospective study. *Acta Paediatr.* 2004 Oct;93(10):1346-8.

[124] Wickes IG. A history of infant feeding. III. Eighteenth and nineteenth century writers. *Arch Dis Child*. 1953 Aug;28(140):332-40.

[125] Dunn PM. Dr William Cadogan (1711-1797) of Bristol and the management of infants. *Arch Dis Child*. 1992 Jan;67(1 Spec No):72-3.

[126] Hunting P. William Cadogan (1711-97): Colossus of child care. *J Med Biogr*. 2011 Nov;19(4):182-3.

[127] Moscucci O. The Science of Woman: Gynaecology and Gender in England, 1800-1929. Cambridge: Cambridge University Press; 1990.

[128] Dunn PM. *George Armstrong MD (1719-1789) and his dispensary for the infant poor*. Arch Dis Child Fetal Neonatal Ed. 2002 Nov;87(3):F228-31.

[129] Maloney WJ. George and John Armstrong of Castleton. *Two Eighteenth-Century Medical Pioneers*. Edinburgh: E & S Livingstone; 1954.

[130] Fildes V. The English wet-nurse and her role in infant care 1538-1800. *Med Hist*. 1988 Apr;32(2):142-73.

[131] Baines MA. Infant-Alimentation; or, Artificial Feeding, as a Substitute for Breast-Milk, Considered in its Physical and Social Aspects. *Lancet;* 1869.

[132] WHO. The physiological basis of breastfeeding. In: WHO (ed). *Infant and Young Child Feeding: Model Chapter for Textbooks for Medical Students and Allied Health Professionals*. WHO; 2009.

[133] Dewey KG, Nommsen-Rivers LA, Heinig MJ and Cohen RJ. Risk factors for suboptimal infant breastfeeding behavior, delayed onset of lactation, and excess neonatal weight loss. *Pediatrics*. 2003 Sep;112(3 Pt 1):607-19.

[134] Shannon M, King TL and Kennedy HP. Allostasis: A theoretical framework for understanding and evaluating perinatal health outcomes. *J Obstet Gynecol Neonatal Nurs*. 2007 Mar-Apr;36(2):125-34.

[135] Vittner D, McGrath J, Robinson J, Lawhon G, Cusson R, Eisenfeld L, Walsh S, Young E and Cong X. Increase in Oxytocin From Skin-to-Skin Contact Enhances Development of Parent-Infant Relationship. *Biol Res Nurs.* 2018 Jan;20(1):54-62.

[136] Hochberg Z, Feil R, Constancia M, Fraga M, Junien C, Carel JC, Boileau P, Le Bouc Y, Deal CL, Lillycrop K, Scharfmann R, Sheppard A, Skinner M, Szyf M, Waterland RA, Waxman DJ, Whitelaw E, Ong K and Albertsson-Wikland K. Child health, developmental plasticity, and epigenetic programming. *Endocr Rev.* 2011 Apr;32(2):159-224.

[137] Neovita Study Group. Timing of initiation, patterns of breastfeeding, and infant survival: Prospective analysis of pooled data from three randomised trials. *Lancet Glob Health.* 2016 Apr;4(4):e266-75.

[138] Moore ER, Bergman N, Anderson GC and Medley N. Early skin-to-skin contact for mothers and their healthy newborn infants. *Cochrane Database Syst Rev.* 2016 Nov 25;11:CD003519.

[139] UNICEF. *Global database on Infant and Young Child Feeding.* New York: UNICEF; 2018.

[140] Takahashi K, Ganchimeg T, Ota E, Vogel JP, Souza JP, Laopaiboon M, Castro CP, Jayaratne K, Ortiz-Panozo E, Lumbiganon P and Mori R. Prevalence of early initiation of breastfeeding and determinants of delayed initiation of breastfeeding: Secondary analysis of the WHO Global Survey. *Sci Rep.* 2017 Mar 21;7:44868.

[141] Patel A, Bucher S, Pusdekar Y, Esamai F, Krebs NF, Goudar SS, Chomba E, Garces A, Pasha O, Saleem S, Kodkany BS, Liechty EA, Kodkany B, Derman RJ, Carlo WA, Hambidge K, Goldenberg RL, Althabe F, Berrueta M, Moore JL, McClure EM, Koso-Thomas M and Hibberd PL. Rates and determinants of early initiation of breastfeeding and exclusive breast feeding at 42 days postnatal in six low and middle-income countries: A prospective cohort study. *Reprod Health.* 2015 Jun 8;12 Suppl 2:S10.

[142] Gao H, Wang Q, Hormann E, Stuetz W, Stiller C, Biesalski HK and Scherbaum V. Breastfeeding practices on postnatal wards in urban

and rural areas of the Deyang region, Sichuan province of China. *Int Breastfeed J.* 2016;11:11.

[143] WHO. Exclusive breastfeeding for optimal growth, development and health of infants. *e-Library of Evidence for Nutrition Actions (eLENA)* 2018 [cited; Available from: http://www.who.int/elena/titles/exclusive_breastfeeding/en/

[144] Kramer MS and Kakuma R. Optimal duration of exclusive breastfeeding. *Cochrane Database Syst Rev.* 2012;8:CD003517.

[145] Kramer MS, Matush L, Vanilovich I, Platt RW, Bogdanovich N, Sevkovskaya Z, Dzikovich I, Shishko G, Collet JP, Martin RM, Davey Smith G, Gillman MW, Chalmers B, Hodnett E and Shapiro S. Effects of prolonged and exclusive breastfeeding on child height, weight, adiposity, and blood pressure at age 6.5 y: Evidence from a large randomized trial. *Am J Clin Nutr.* 2007 Dec;86(6):1717-21.

[146] UNICEF. *The State of the World's Children 2017: Children in a Digital World.* New York: UNICEF; 2017.

[147] Obladen M. From swill milk to certified milk: Progress in cow's milk quality in the 19th century. *Ann Nutr Metab.* 2014;64(1):80-7.

[148] Faruque AS, Mahalanabis D, Islam A, Hoque SS and Hasnat A. Breast feeding and oral rehydration at home during diarrhoea to prevent dehydration. *Arch Dis Child.* 1992 Aug;67(8):1027-9.

[149] WHO. *Declaration of Alma-Ata. International Conference on Primary Health Care, Alma-Ata, USSR,* 6-12 September 1978 Geneva: WHO; 1978.

[150] WHO. Integrated management of childhood illness: Conclusions. WHO Division of Child Health and Development. *Bull World Health Organ.* 1997;75 Suppl 1:119-28.

[151] Gwatkin DR. *The current state of knowledge about targeting health programs to reach the poor.* New York: World Bank; 2000.

[152] Victora CG, Wagstaff A, Armstrong Schellenberg J, Gwatkin D, Claeson M and Habicht JP. Applying an equity lens to child health and mortality: More of the same is not enough. *Lancet.* 2003;362(9379):233-41.

[153] Amir LH. ABM clinical protocol #4: Mastitis, revised March 2014. *Breastfeed Med.* 2014 Jun;9(5):239-43.

[154] Hahn-Holbrook J, Dunkel Schettler C and Haselton M. Breastfeeding and Maternal Mental and Physical Health. In: Spiers M, Geller P and Kloss J (eds). *Women's health psychology.* New Jersey: Wiley; 2013. p. 414-39.

[155] van den Engel-Hoek L, van Hulst KC, van Gerven MH, van Haaften L and de Groot SA. Development of oral motor behavior related to the skill assisted spoon feeding. *Infant Behav Dev.* 2014 May;37(2):187-91.

[156] McKinney CM, Glass RP, Coffey P, Rue T, Vaughn MG and Cunningham M. Feeding Neonates by Cup: A Systematic Review of the Literature. *Matern Child Health J.* 2016 Aug;20(8):1620-33.

[157] Dewey KG. *Guiding principles for complementary feeding of the breastfed child.* Washington: PAHO, WHO; 2003.

[158] Cone TE. History of Infant feeding. From the earliest years through the development of scientific concepts. In: Bond JT (ed). *Infant and Child Feeding.* New York: Academic Press; 1981. p. 4-34.

[159] Schuman AJ. A concise history of infant formula (twists and turns included). *Contemp Pediatrics.* 2003;20:91-103.

[160] Grabmayr S and Scherbaum V. Ernährungsformen in den ersten Lebenstagen (Forms of nutrition in the first few days of life). In: Scherbaum V, Kretschmer U and Perl FM (eds). *Stillen, Frühkindliche Ernährung und reproduktive Gesundheit [Breastfeeding, Early Childhood Nutrition and Reproductive Health].* Köln: Deutscher Ärzte-Verlag; 2003. p. 71-4.

[161] Barness LA. History of infant feeding practices. *Am J Clin Nutr.* 1987 Jul;46(1 Suppl):168-70.

[162] Krasselt A, Scherbaum V and Tönz O. Muttermilchersatzprodukte (Breastmilk substitute products). In: Scherbaum V, Perl FM and Kretschmer U (eds). *Stillen, Frühkindliche Ernährung und reproduktive Gesundheit. [Breastfeeding, Early Childhood Nutrition and Reproductive Health].* Köln: Deutscher Ärzte-Verlag; 2003. p. 14-24.

[163] Routh CHF. *Infant feeding and its influence on Life or the Causes and Prevention of Infant Mortality.* New York: William Wood; 1879.

[164] Schwab MG. Mechanical Milk. An Essay on the Social History of Infant Formula. *Childhood.* 1996;3:479-99.

[165] Soxhlet F. Die chemischen Unterschiede zwischen Kuh- und Frauenmilch und die Mittel zu ihrer Ausgleichung (The chemical differences between cow's and human milk and the means to equalize them) *Münchener Medizinische Wochenschrift.* 1893;40: 61-5.

[166] Wood AL. The history of artificial feeding of infants. *J Am Diet Assoc.* 1955 May;31(5):474-82.

[167] Mepham TB. "Humanizing" milk: The formulation of artificial feeds for infants (1850-1910). *Med Hist.* 1993 Jul;37(3):225-49.

[168] Rotch TM. An historical scetch of the development of percentage feeding. *NY Med J* 1907;85:532-40.

[169] Rosenstern I. Heinrich Finkelstein, 1865-1942. *J Pediatr.* 1956 Oct;49(4):499-503.

[170] Koletzko B, Baker S, Cleghorn G, Neto UF, Gopalan S, Hernell O, Hock QS, Jirapinyo P, Lonnerdal B, Pencharz P, Pzyrembel H, Ramirez-Mayans J, Shamir R, Turck D, Yamashiro Y and Zong-Yi D. Global standard for the composition of infant formula: Recommendations of an ESPGHAN coordinated international expert group. *J Pediatr Gastroenterol Nutr.* 2005 Nov;41(5):584-99.

[171] Krasselt A and Scherbaum V. Selbstherstellung von Säuglingsmilch. (Home-made infant formula) In: Scherbaum V, Kretschmer U and Perl FM (eds). *Stillen, Frühkindliche Ernährung und reproduktive Gesundheit. (Breastfeeding, Early Childhood Nutrition and Reproductive Health)* Köln: Deutscher Ärzte-Verlag; 2003. p. 25-31.

[172] WHO. *International Code of Marketing of Breast-Milk Substitutes.* Geneva: WHO; 1981.

[173] Cattaneo A. The benefits of breastfeeding or the harm of formula feeding? *J Paediatr Child Health.* 2008 Jan;44(1-2):1-2.

[174] Scherbaum V. Säuglingsernährung in Nordirak. (Infant feeding in Northern Iraq) *ErnährungsUmschau.* 2003;50(12):476-80.
[175] Ho TF, Yip WC, Tay JS and Wong HB. Variability in osmolality of home prepared formula milk samples. *J Trop Pediatr.* 1985 Apr;31(2):92-4.
[176] Barennes H, Andriatahina T, Latthaphasavang V, Anderson M and Srour LM. Misperceptions and misuse of Bear Brand coffee creamer as infant food: National cross sectional survey of consumers and paediatricians in Laos. *BMJ.* 2008;337:a1379.
[177] Slesak G, Douangdala P, Inthalad S, Onekeo B, Somsavad S, Sisouphanh B, Srour LM and Barennes H. *Misuse of coffee creamer as a breast milk substitute: A lethal case revealing high use in an ethnic minority village in Northern Laos.* . BMJ; 2009.
[178] Newton ER. Breastmilk: The gold standard. *Clin Obstet Gynecol.* 2004 Sep;47(3):632-42.
[179] Ballard O and Morrow AL. Human milk composition: Nutrients and bioactive factors. *Pediatr Clin North Am.* 2013 Feb;60(1):49-74.
[180] Strauss LG (ed). *Disease in Milk - The Remedy Pasteurisation.* New York: Dutton; 1913.
[181] Jelliffe DB and Jelliffe EFP. *Human Milk in the Modern World. Psychosocial, Nutritional, and Economic Significance.* Oxford: Oxford University Press; 1979.
[182] Radbill SX. Infant feeding through ages. *Clin Pediatr (Phila).* 1981;20:613-21.
[183] Dwork D. The milk option. An aspect of the history of the infant welfare movement in England 1898-1908. *Med Hist.* 1987 Jan;31(1):51-69.
[184] Lee KS. Infant mortality decline in the late 19th and early 20th centuries: The role of market milk. *Perspect Biol Med.* 2007 Autumn;50(4):585-602.
[185] Exner M, Hartemann P and Kistemann T. Hygiene and health - the need for a holistic approach. *Am J Infect Control.* 2001 Aug;29(4):228-31.

[186] Bloomfield SF and Scott EA. Developing an effective policy for home hygiene: A risk-based approach. *Int J Environ Health Res.* 2003 Jun;13 Suppl 1:S57-66.

[187] Wolf JH. "They Lacked the Right Food": A Brief History of Breastfeeding and the Quest for Social Justice. *J Hum Lact.* 2018 May;34(2):226-31.

[188] Toubas L. Forgotten Lessons of the Past. 100 years after the creation of the first clinic for nurslings. *Biography of Pierre Budin 1846-1907:* University of Oclahoma; 2000.

[189] Dunn PM. Professor Pierre Budin (1846-1907) of Paris, and modern perinatal care. *Archives of Disease in Childhood;* 1995. p. 193-5.

[190] Rollet C. Childhood Mortality in High Risk Groups: Some Methodological Reflections based on French Experience. In: Corsini CA and Viazzo PP (eds). *The Decline of Infant and Child Mortality. The European Experience 1750-1990.* Cambridge: Kluwer Law and Taxation Publisher; 1997. p. 213-27.

[191] Dunn PM. *Stephane Tarnier (1828-1897), the architect of perinatology in France.* Arch Dis Child Fetal Neonatal Ed. 2002 Mar;86(2):F137-9.

[192] Budin P. *The Nursling. The Feeding and Hygiene of Premature and Full-Term Infants.* Authorized Translation by W.J. Maloney. London: Caxton; 1907.

[193] Baker JP. The incubator and the medical discovery of the premature infant. *J Perinatol.* 2000 Jul-Aug;20(5):321-8.

[194] Schneider WH. Puericulture, and the style of French eugenics. *Hist Philos Life Sci.* 1986;8(2):265-77.

[195] Weaver LT. In the balance: Weighing babies and the birth of the infant welfare clinic. *Bull Hist Med.* 2010 Spring;84(1):30-57.

[196] *Mothers and Medicine: A Social History of Infant Feeding, 1890-1950.* Madison, WI. University of Wisconsin Press; 1988.

[197] *Breastfeeding and Media. Exploring Conflicting Discourses That Threaten Public Health.* Cham, Switzerland: Palgrave Macmillan; 2017.

[198] *Save the babies. American public health reform and the prevention of infant mortality 1850-1929.* Ann Arbor: The University of Michigan Press; 1990.

[199] Wolf JH. *Don't kill your baby: Public health and the decline of breastfeeding in the Nineteenth and Twentieth centuries.* Columbus: The Ohio State University Press; 2001.

[200] Koven S and Michel S. Womenly duties: Maternalist politics and the origin of welfare states in France, Germany and Great Britain, and the United States, 1880-1920 *The American Historical review.* 1990;95(4):1076-108.

[201] Richard SA, Black RE, Gilman RH, Guerrant RL, Kang G, Lanata CF, Molbak K, Rasmussen ZA, Sack RB, Valentiner-Branth P and Checkley W. Catch-up growth occurs after diarrhea in early childhood. *J Nutr.* 2014 Jun;144(6):965-71.

[202] Nandi A. *Impact of leave policies on breastfeeding & child health.* Penang, Malaysia: Waba; 2015.

[203] CDC. *Support for Breastfeeding at the workplace.* Atlanta: CDC; 2013.

[204] Liu L, Johnson HL, Cousens S, Perin J, Scott S, Lawn JE, Rudan I, Campbell H, Cibulskis R, Li M, Mathers C and Black RE. Global, regional, and national causes of child mortality: An updated systematic analysis for 2010 with time trends since 2000. *Lancet.* 2012 Jun 9;379(9832):2151-61.

[205] Liu L, Oza S, Hogan D, Chu Y, Perin J, Zhu J, Lawn JE, Cousens S, Mathers C and Black RE. Global, regional, and national causes of under-5 mortality in 2000-15: An updated systematic analysis with implications for the Sustainable Development Goals. *Lancet.* 2016 Dec 17;388(10063):3027-35.

[206] Howson CP, Kinney MV, McDougall L and Lawn JE. Born too soon: Preterm birth matters. *Reprod Health.* 2013;10 Suppl 1:S1.

[207] O'Brien K, Robson K, Bracht M, Cruz M, Lui K, Alvaro R, da Silva O, Monterrosa L and Narvey M. Effectiveness of Family Integrated Care in neonatal intensive care units on infant and parent outcomes:

A multicentre, multinational, cluster-randomised controlled trial. *The Lancet, Child & Adolescent Health.* 2018;2 (4):245–54.

[208] Brockway M, Benzies KM, Carr E and Aziz K. Breastfeeding self-efficacy and breastmilk feeding for moderate and late preterm infants in the Family Integrated Care trial: A mixed methods protocol. *Int Breastfeed J.* 2018;13:29.

[209] Lawn JE, Davidge R, Paul VK, von Xylander S, de Graft Johnson J, Costello A, Kinney MV, Segre J and Molyneux L. Born too soon: Care for the preterm baby. *Reprod Health.* 2013;10 Suppl 1:S5.

[210] Foster JP, Psaila K and Patterson T. Non-nutritive sucking for increasing physiologic stability and nutrition in preterm infants. *Cochrane Database Syst Rev.* 2016 Oct 4;10:CD001071.

[211] Puthussery S, Chutiyami M, Tseng PC, Kilby L and Kapadia J. Effectiveness of early intervention programs for parents of preterm infants: A meta-review of systematic reviews. *BMC Pediatr.* 2018 Jul 9;18(1):223.

[212] Conde-Agudelo A and Diaz-Rossello JL. Kangaroo mother care to reduce morbidity and mortality in low birthweight infants. *Cochrane Database Syst Rev.* 2016 Aug 23(8):CD002771.

[213] Arshiya S, Khaleeq UR and Manjula SM. Clinical update and treatment of lactation insufficiency. *Medical Journal of Islamic World Academy of Sciences.* 2013;21(1):19-28.

[214] Kent G. *Breastfeeding - a human rights issue?* London and New Delhi: The Society for International Development; 2001.

In: New Research on Breastfeeding ...
Editor: Kai Santos Melo

ISBN: 978-1-53617-061-0
© 2020 Nova Science Publishers, Inc.

Chapter 5

USE OF BREAST MILK AND BREASTFEEDING AS A NON PHARMACOLOGICAL METHOD FOR PROCEDURAL PAIN MANAGEMENT

Ayşe Şener Taplak and Sevinç Polat, PhD
RN. Department of Pediatric Nursing,
Yozgat Bozok University, Yozgat, Turkey

ABSTRACT

Newborns and infants require needle-related painful procedures for scheduled childhood immunizations, as well as medical procedures performed for diagnostic and treatment purposes during the course of childhood illnesses. Uncontrolled pain causes clinical instability as a result of development of complications such as changes in heart rate, respiratory rate, blood pressure, intracranial pressure, oxygen saturation along with intraventricular hemorrhaging. Recurrent pain experienced for the purpose of diagnosis and treatment leads to atrophy in the brain of the infant, which can result in neurodevelopmental problems and a decrease in the subcortical white and gray matter in the brain.

The prevention or minimization of pain is the right of any newborns and infants. As infants experience a healthy neonatal period when their pain is under control, their duration of stay in hospital is reduced and their growth and development can accelerate, which contributes positively to the national economy. However, studies on pain in infants reveal that 40-60% of infants do not receive any preventive or therapeutic application during painful procedures. In recognizing the adverse consequences of untreated pain in infants, national guidelines for evidence informed pain assessment and management practices have been developed. An intervention recommended in such guidelines for procedural pain management is breastmilk and breastfeeding.

This study is aimed to provide an updated synthesis of the current state of the evidence for the effectiveness of breastfeeding and breast milk feeding in reducing procedural pain in preterm and full-term born infants. A systematic search of key electronic databases (PubMed, Science Direct, Google Scholar) will be sought. The main criteria are behavioral or physiological indicators and compound pain scores and other clinically important results reported by the authors.

The findings of the studies show that breastfeeding is more effective in reducing pain during painful interventions such as heel lance, aspiration and vaccination in newborns and infants, compared to studies using breast milk or breast milk smell alone.

Keywords: breast milk, breastfeeding, pain management, infant, newborn

INTRODUCTION

Examined as the fifth vital sign; pain is defined as an unpleasant biochemical and emotional condition or behavior, which arises from a certain area of the body, develops depending on an actual or potential tissue damage, and is affected by the person's past experiences (Aliefendioglu, 2015). Pain transduction pathways are ready during labor and transmit painful stimuli to the pain center in the brain even if they are immature (Walker, 2014). Thus, preterm and term infants show a behavioral, psychological and hormonal response to pain (Maxwell, Malavolta, Fraga, 2013; Anand, 2017).

Some studies on animals and neonates have reported that the responses infants display toward painful stimuli in repeated and prolonged episodes may lead to long-term outcomes as well as adverse effects on neurologic and behavioral development (Morais et al., 2016; Young, 2005). This is because the pain develops at a critical time of neurologic maturation (Witt et al., 2016). Granau, reported evidences indicating long-term associations among repeated pain in the Neonatal Intensive Care Unit (NICU) and altered brain development, neuro-development, programming of stress systems and late pain perception in preterm infants (Granau, 2013). Preterm infants are under a higher risk in terms of developmental disabilities. Cerebral palsy, hyperactivity, and specific learning disabilities are the most common types of these disabilities (Standley and Swedberg, 2011). In term infants, on the other hand, pain has a negative effect on family-infant interaction, infant's adaptation to the outer world, behaviors, diet and growth and may cause differences in the development of the brain and senses (Vinall et al., 2012; Akcan and Polat, 2017). In addition, repeated pain episodes may differentiate the pain threshold in children and the distress and phobic reactions caused by needle procedures may affect the child's pain memory and obstruct the completion of the next procedures (Hamilton 1995; Fitzgerald and Walker 2006; Noel et al., 2012).

Today, infants still experience pain ranging from moderate to severe levels in the hospital environment (Derebent, 2006; Stevens et al., 2014; Twycross et al., 2013). Studies on pain have revealed that 40-60% of infants do not receive any preventive or therapeutic administration during painful procedures (Carbajal et al., 2008; Lago et al., 2005; Bellieni et al., 2017). An extensive prospective study conducted in France in 2008 revealed that while specific pharmacological or non-pharmacological analgesia was administered to only 21% of infants before painful procedures and the ongoing analgesia was administered at the rate of 34% (Carbajal et al., 2008).

It is every child's right to lead a pain-free life. Thus, pain management and treatment in children is an ethical obligation (Derebent, 2006; Akcan and Polat, 2017). Primary purposes of care include killing the pain and enhancing comfort and life quality as from infancy. Many non-pharmacological methods are used in the pain management for infants (Akcan and Polat, 2016; Küçük Alemdar and Kardaş Özdemir 2017; Tekgündüz et al., 2019). Among these methods, breast milk and breastfeeding are primarily preferred in coping with the pain because they do not require a special preparation and are more economic and natural (Uğurlu, 2017). The first contact between the mother and infant generally occurs with the mother's breast. The infant considers its mother's breast not only an organ providing a nutritional source, but also an indivisible part of its own body. Breastfeeding is a whole including sensual contact, mother-infant communication and sense of taste and breast milk is an analgesic. Breastfeeding activates sense receptors and sense of taste in the infant's skin. Besides, fats, proteins and other nutrients in breast milk stop the transmission of sense of pain by stimulating opioids and blocking pain fibers that lead to the spinal cord and thus, they show an analgesic effect (Gray, Miller, Phillip & Blass, 2002; Dilli, Küçük & Dallar, 2009). In numerous studies, it has been revealed that breast milk, besides its common benefits, is effective on reducing pain that develops during minor painful procedures such as heel lance, vaccination and aspiration in newborns and infants (Hsieh et al., 2018; Ou-Yang et al., 2013; Özdogan et al., 2010).

METHODS

This study is aimed to provide an updated synthesis of the current state of the evidence for the effectiveness of breastfeeding and breast milk feeding in reducing procedural pain in preterm and full-term infants. A systematic search of key electronic databases (PubMed, Science Direct, Google Scholar) will be sought. The main criterias are behavioral or physiological indicators and composite pain scores, as well as other clinically important outcomes reported by the authors included studies.

Pain Factors in Newborns and Infants

In various epidemiological studies on interventional procedures that cause pain in newborns and infants; procedure types and number of painful procedures are discussed (Table 1).

Table 1. The study findings concerning the number and type of painful interventions applied to newborns

Author	Gestational age GA (week)	Number of painful interventions	The most frequently applied intervention
Baker and Rutter, 1995	N = 54, (GA) = 23-41	A total of 3000 interventions in 3 months. 74% of the newborns are younger than 31st gestational week.	Heel lance procedure (56%) and endotracheal aspiration (26%)
Zahr and Balian, 1995	N = 55, GA = 23-32	14-25 interventions a day or 273 interventions within 2 weeks per infant (Including daily activities like changing diapers and weighing).	Respectively; aspiration, heel lance procedure, putting on an intravenous cannula, giving position/changing diapers
Johnston et al., 1997	N = 239, GA = 23-42	2134 interventions (1.99 interventions a day or 28 interventions within 2 weeks per infant).	Application of inserting an intravenous (IV) cannula following heel lance procedure
Stevens et al., 2003	N = 194, GA = 27-31;	10 interventions a day or 140 interventions within 2 weeks per infant. Most of the interventions were performed on high-risk newborns.	Aspiration, heel lance procedure, and insertion of an intravenous cannula
Simons et al., 2003	N = 151, GA = 25-42	19.674 interventions within 1375 days (14.3 interventions a day or 200 interventions within 2 weeks); 31% of which are repeated interventions.	Aspiration (63%) and heel lance procedure
Carbajal et al., 2008	N = 430, GA = 24-42	60.969 interventions within 2 weeks (12 interventions a day or 168 interventions within 2 weeks per infant).	Aspiration (28%) and heel lance procedure (19%)
Cignacco et al, 2009	N = 120, GA = 24-27	38.626 interventions within the first 14 days (17.3 interventions a day or 242 interventions within 2 weeks).	Continuous Positive Airway Pressure-CPAP (26%) Manipulation and heel lance procedure (17%)
Johnston et al., 2011	N = 582 GA = 28-36	3508 interventions causing tissue damage and 14.085 interventions not causing tissue damage within 1 week.	Among interventions causing tissue damage, the most frequently applied procedure was heel lance procedure and among interventions not causing tissue damage, the most frequently applied procedure was tracheal aspiration.

In the study conducted by Barker to determine the frequency and type of procedures applied in Neonatale Intensive Care Unıt (NICU), it was determined that heel lance was the most frequently performed invasive intervention (Barker and Rutter, 1995). In another study, it was also found that the second most painful procedure was endotracheal aspiration (Cignacco, 2006). As cited by Cignacco, in a study conducted in the Swiss clinics, it was determined that averagely 4092 procedures were performed on 11 intubated newborns within the first 14 days of their lives and 64.8% of these procedures were related with intubated preterm infants younger than 28th gestational week. In the same study, it was found that a preterm infant was exposed to 372 painful procedures a day within the first 14 days of its life on average (Cignacco, 2006). Besides these procedures, diagnostic interventions such as arterial catheter application, bronchoscopy, endoscopy, lumbar puncture, retinopathy or preterm examination and venous blood sampling and therapeutic interventions such as insertion/removal of a urinary catheter, central catheter, chest tube, gavage tube, peripheric venous catheter and tracheal intubation tube, intramuscular injection, mechanical ventilation, postural drainage and taking out plasters; and surgical procedures such as circumcision are among painful interventions for newborns (Britto et al., 2014; Ceuz, Fernandes and Oliveira, 2016). Table 1 shows the study findings concerning the number and type of painful interventions applied to newborns.

THE EFFECTS OF PAIN AND PAIN RESPONSE IN NEWBORNS/INFANTS

The pain experienced by newborns and infants due to the stressful intensive care environment and invasive interventions they are exposed to affects the clinical course of their illnesses, infants' adaptation to the outer world, their behaviors, family-infant interaction, feeding, growth, development of brain and senses negatively (Dinçer, 2011; Törüner and

Büyükgönenç, 2017; Akcan and Polat, 2017). The most sensitive cell populations in the brain of preterm infants to damage are subplate neurons and preoligodendrocytes. The pain experienced due to repeated interventions may cause apoptosis and excitotoxicity in subplate neurons as a result of excessive release of glutamate and excessive diffusion of calcium into neurons (Talos et al., 2006). Neonatal pain stress affects preoligodendrocytes covering axones before transforming into axones which produce myelin. Immaturity of these cells makes them sensitive to especially oxygen and nitrogen types and to cytokines released from microgliads. The pain experienced depending on an interventional

Table 2. Short and long term effects of pain

Short term	Effects
Tachycardia	May cause changes in the intracranial blood volume and cerebral hemorrhage.
Partial decrease of O_2 pressure	May cause intraventricular and ventricular hemorrhages.
Increase in the β-endorphin level Normal: 10-27 pg/ml	May cause neurological dysfunctions.
Diaphragmatic spasm	Important changes in the intrathoracic pressure may significantly affect intracranial pressure and cerebral blood flow and cause intraventricular hemorrhage.
Long term	Effects
Increase in the O2 consumption, heart rate and blood pressure	During the pain, there might be overload and hemorrhage in weak and immature veins depending on the increase in O2 consumption, heart rate, and blood pressure.
Deterioration in the glucose balance	In infants, a serious and long term hyperglycemia develops in case of pain due to deterioration in the glucose balance and then hypoglycemia can observe as a result of the discharge of carbohydrate and fat stores.
Increase in the protein breakdown	During pain, growth and development break down due to the increase in the protein breakdown.
Increase in the cortisol secretion	Increased cortisol secretion deteriorates the immune system of the preterm infant, suppresses anabolic formation, shrinks muscles, reduces insulin sensitivity, and affects growth negatively.
Sensitivity to pain	Hypersensitivity to pain develops in newborns exposed to repeated painful stimuli. The infant gives a greater response to pain during the next pain experiences than the expected. Hypersensitivity increases cortisol secretion and causes longer and more intense pain responses.

procedure may pause the development of pre-myelinating cells by inducing both oxidative stress and inflammatory reactions (Buntinx et al., 2004; Slater et al., 2012).

Table 2 summarizes many other effects caused by pain in newborns in the short and long term (Zempsky et al., 2003; Akcan and Polat, 2017; Çöçelli and Bacaksız, 2008).

As newborns and infants are unable to express their pain verbally, they develop physiological, behavioral and hormonal responses to pain (Beltramini et al., 2017). Responses to pain are evaluated as:

1. *Physiological response:* It is reported that the most frequent physiological responses are the increased heart rate, blood pressure and respiration rate, decreased O_2 saturation, paleness or redness, sweating, and pupil dilation (Ballweg 2007; Diego et al., 2009; Padhye et al., 2009).
2. *Behavioral response:* Facial and body movements are evaluated as behavioral responses to pain.
   - *Facial Movements:* the most studied one among motor signs is changes in the facial expression. The most frequent changes are frowning eyebrows, squinting or closing in the eyes, broad nasal bridge, and changes in the shape of the mouth like curling of the lips. These facial expressions observed depending on pain are not so apparent in preterm infants (Walter et al., 2010).
   - *Body Movements:* Bodily responses such as opening the hands, squeezing the fists, protecting a part of the body, restlessness, turning the head from one side to the other, rubbing the back, jumping and kicking are observed (Williams et al., 2009; Blount and Loiselle, 2009).
3. *Hormonal and catabolic stress response:* Plasma renin activity, catecholamine levels (epinephrine, norepinephrine), cortisol levels, nitrogen excretion, growth hormone, glucagon, aldosterone secretion, glucose, lactate, pyruvate, ketone, the increase in the serum levels of non-esterified fatty acids, and the decrease in

insulin secretion are observed (Henry et al., 2004; Grunau et al., 2004). It has been reported that chest physiotherapy and endotracheal aspiration cause significant increases in plasma epinephrine and norepinephrine levels in preterm infants receiving ventilation treatment (Krishnan, 2013; Moultrie, Slater, Hartley, 2017). Table 3 shows systemic effects of pain.

Table 3. Systemic effects of pain

Systems	Effects of Pain
Cardiovascular System	– Tachycardia – Systemic hypertension – Increase in the cardiac output – Increase in the afterload and the heart's work load – Increase in the heart's need for oxygen (Dunwoody et al., 2008; Brand & Canchi, 2013).
Respiratory System	– Tachypnea/Respiratory alkalosis – Reduced vital capacity and expansion/atelectasis and hypoxia risk in the lungs – Reduced alveolar ventilation/hypoxia – Failure of spitting out secretions due to poor coughing and the risk of infection and hypoxia (Dikmen, 2012; Brand & Canchi, 2013).
Gastrointestinal System	– Reduced gastric discharge and motility – Reduced oral intake – Nausea and vomiting (Brand & Canchi, 2013).
Endocrine System	– Increase in the stress response and stress hormones – Deterioration in the gluconeogenesis, glycogenolysis, hypercalcemia, and lucose tolerance – Negative nitrogen balance (Brand & Canchi, 2013).
Genitourinary System	Increase in the antidiuretic hormone level, reduced urination, sodium, and water retention (Brand & Canchi, 2013; Erdine, 2007).
Nervous System	– Procedural pain hinders the development of unmyelinated cells by inducing both oxidative stress and inflammatory reaction (Brummelte et al., 2012; Slater et al., 2010; Hansson, 2006; Anand et al., 2007; Perrone et al., 2017). – Repeated painful stimuli affect the brain development negatively and cause lower cognitive and neurological development in the following periods. The risk of intraventricular hemorrhage increases depending on the increase of intracranial pressure (Vinall & Grunau, 2014; Grunau, 2013; Ranger et al., 2013).
Hematologic System	-Hypercoagulation (Brand & Canchi, 2013).
Immune System	Deterioration in the immune response and decrease in the tissue healing (Brand and Canchi, 2013).

Pain Assessment

Pain in neonatal and infancy periods is assessed conducting validity and reliability studies and using standardized scales. These scales used are multidimensional and broad pain assessment tools that are specific to acute or chronic pain and address physiological and behavioral changes (Roofhooft, 2014). The most frequently used scales in newborns and infants are "Premature Infant Pain Profile- PIPP and Premature Infant Pain Profile Revised-PIPP-R", "Neonatal Face Coding System,-NFCS", "Neonatal Infant Pain Scale,-NIPS", "Neonatal Postoperative Pain Scale-CRIES", and "Face, Legs, Activity, Cry, Consolability- FLACC" (Stevens et al., 2014; Witt, Coynor, Edwards, & Bradshaw, 2016).

The Use of Breast Milk and Breastfeeding in Pain Management

The most effective approaches for pain control are raising awareness about the presence of pain in newborns, minimize invasive interventions applied to infants as much as possible and minimize pain in inevitable cases by means of pharmacological and non-pharmacological methods (Yigit, Ecevit & Koroglu, 2015). It is reported that breastfeeding is an approach that should be preferred first even in minor painful interventions in newborns. It has been found that giving breast milk via a dropper, feeding bottle or an injector in cases where breastfeeding is not possible (in case of mother's absence or breastfeeding difficulties) is also effective on painful procedures. In addition, it is stated that for every newborn, the breast milk of his/her own mother is more effective (Reece-Stremtan et al., 2016). It is thought that the effect of lactose which is a disaccharide on the oral sense of taste and the correlation of endogenous opiate pathways with each other are effective on the analgesic effect of breast milk. This perception of taste is well-developed even in preterm infants (Gibbins and Stevens, 2001). Thus, breast milk containing tryptophan increases beta-endorphin and reduces pain (Barrett, Kent & Voudouris, 2000; Blass, 1997). Analgesic efficiency of breast milk was demonstrated in rats by Blass & Fitzgerald in 1988 for the first time. In the same study, it was concluded that this effect which could be obstructed with naltrexone occurred on the basis of opioids (Blass and Fitzgerald, 1988). Afterwards, it was found that breast milk had an antinociceptive effect on newborns and this effect could be associated with not only the taste factor, but also with fat and protein components (Blass, 1997).

In this section, studies on breastfeeding, breast milk and breast milk smell were scanned on the databases of Pubmed, Sciencedirect and Google Scholar and the relevant titles were presented in tables.

BREASTFEEDING

After realizing the adverse outcomes of untreated pain in preterm and term infants, various guidelines have been developed in order to assess and manage pain in the light of evidences (AAP, 2016; Yigit, Ecevit & Koroglu, 2015). In these guidelines, one of the practices recommended for interventional pain management is breastfeeding. The latest synthesis of evidences indicating that breastfeeding or expressed breast milk is used as a pain relief method in infants was published in a Cochrane review in 2012. In this context, Shah et al., examined 20 studies examining a total of 2071 newborns. Studies using direct breastfeeding (10 studies, n = 1075) or expressed breast milk (10 studies, n = 996) during painful procedures associated with acute needle such as venipuncture, heel lance and intramuscular injections were compared (Shah et al., 2012). The other 10 studies using direct breastfeeding had similar results indicating that breastfeeding had a therapeutic effect on physiological findings and crying duration. In addition, the results showed that there was a significant decrease in pain scores in the measurements which were performed using standard pain scales such as PIPP Scores, Douleur Aiguë du Nouveau-né (DAN) Scores, Neonatal Infant Pain Scale (NIPS), and Neonatal Facial Coding System (NFCS) Scores (Shah et al., 2012). In other relevant studies, it was reported that heart rate, duration of crying, duration of first crying, and total duration of crying were significantly lower in breastfed newborns than newborns who were swaddled and held by their mothers or received oral sucrose, pacifier, placebo during the procedure or were not intervened at all (Gray, 2002; Gradin et al., 2004; Philips et al., 2005; Codipietro et al., 2008; Weissman et al., 2009; Okan et al., 2010; Efe and Ozer, 2007). Table 4 shows the results of current studies using breastfeeding during painful procedures.

EXPRESSED BREAST MILK

The most natural non-pharmacological method for pain control in newborns during mild and moderate painful procedures is breastfeeding. However, the mother may not be present in the unit or may not want to witness her infant suffer during painful interventions.

The best alternative to breastfeeding is expressed breast milk, but the effective dose interval of expressed breast milk has not been determined yet. In the light of the studies; 2-5 mL expressed breast milk can be given, preferably as hindmilk, before interventions causing mild and moderate pain. On the other hand, the effectiveness of this approach in repeated painful interventions has not been investigated, yet (Yigit, Ecevit & Koroglu, 2015). In the relevant studies, various amounts of expressed breast milk were applied to newborns or infants via an injector or a dropper. These studies include the ones comparing breast milk with placebo and also with other non-pharmacological pain relief methods. Expressed breast milk reduced the duration of crying compared to placebo and the behavioral pain response which was measured using the NFCS in comparison to placebo reduced in one of the three studies reporting this result (Skogsdal et al., 1997; Ors et al., 1999; Bucher et al., 2000; Jatana, Dalal & Wilson, 2003; Uyan et al., 2005; Mathai, Natrajan & Rajalakshmi, 2006; Özdoğan et al., 2010; Upadhyay et al., 2004). In some studies, on the other hand, it was found that breast milk was less effective on reducing oral sucrose in 12.5%, 20% and 25% concentrations; oral glucose, use of pacifier and rocking in 25% and 30% concentrations; duration of crying and heart rate, compared to the control groups (Blass and Miller, 2001; Ozdogan et al., 2010; Skogsdal, Eriksson & Schollin, 1997; Ors et al., 1999; Yilmaz and Arikan, 2011; Jatana, Dalal & Wilson, 2003; Mathai, Natrajan & Rajalakshmi, 2006). In the initial pain-related studies conducted by giving expressed breast milk, it was found that giving 1-2 ml expressed breast milk two minutes before the heel lance procedure showed no analgesic effectiveness; whereas, giving 5 ml expressed breast milk was effective (Ors et al., 1999; Ozek, Cebeci & Ors, 2001; Upadhyay et al., 2004; Blass and Miller, 2001). This effect of breast milk depending on dose was thought to be associated with fat content (Altun & Ozek, 2005). Regarding this hypothesis, it was showed that giving hindmilk during the heel lance procedure in term infants had an analgesic effectiveness (Altun et al., 2010). However, giving 2 ml standard breast milk in late preterm infants did not show any significant analgesic effectiveness for the same intervention (Bueno et al., 2012). It was reported that giving 2 ml expressed breast milk to term infants two minutes before venous blood sampling caused a significant decrease in their pain responses, as long as there was less than 25% glucose (Sahoo et al., 2013). In a study conducted with preterm infants, giving 5 mL expressed breast milk caused a significant decrease in pain scores following the heel lance procedure, although it did not shorten the duration of crying (Ou-Yang et al., 2013). Table 5 shows the results of the studies using expressed breast milk during painful procedures.

BREAST MILK SMELL

In preterm infants, sense of smell develops after the 26th gestational week and newborns are able to discern smell of their mother's milk even without feeding experience (Jebreili et al., 2015; Rattaz et al., 2005). It is reported that breast milk smell has several positive effects on newborns, such as shortening the duration of hospitalization, calming down infant and reducing pain (Nishitani et al., 2009; Aoyama et al., 2010; Küçük Alemdar and Kardaş Özdemir, 2017).

In their study, Baudesson de Chanville et al., found that breast milk smell was more effective on reducing newborns' pain during venipuncture procedure, compared to the control group (Baudesson de Chanville et al., 2017).

In the study conducted by Kucuk Alemdar and Kardas Ozdemir, to examine the effects of breast milk smell, amniotic fluid smell and mother's smell on pain, physiological parameters and durations of crying in reducing preterm infants' pain during heel lance procedure, they determined that there was no difference between the groups in terms of reducing infants' pain (Küçük Alemdar and Kardaş Özdemir, 2017).

In the study by Akcan and Polat, it was determined that the newborns who smelled breast milk during heel lance procedure felt less pain than the control group. Akcan and Polat, found that the newborns who smelled breast milk, amniotic fluid, and lavender during heel lance procedure had significantly lower NIPS scores during and after heel lance procedure, compared to the control group (Akcan and Polat, 2016).

In the study conducted by Jebreili et al., to compare breast milk smell and vanilla smell during venipuncture procedure in preterm infants, they determined that both of the methods were effective on calming down the infants during the procedure; however, breast milk smell was more effective on calming down them after the procedure (Jebreili et al., 2015).

In their study, Aoyama et al., compared breast milk smell and formula milk smell and determined that breast milk smell increased the oxygenation of blood supply in the orbito-frontal area in newborns, compared to formula milk smell (Aoyama et al., 2010).

In their study, Nishitani et al., compared breast milk smell, another mother's milk smell and formula milk smell during heel lance procedure and found that behavioral responses and saliva cortisol levels of the newborns smelling their own mothers' milk smell were significantly lower than others and they had less pain (Nishitani et al., 2009).

Table 4. Studies Using Breastfeeding During Painful Procedures

Authors	Procedure	Method	Groups	Measurement	Results
Gad et al., 2019	Routine immunizations 120 infants	Randomized controlled experimental trial	Breastfeeding group Sucrose group Control group	The FLACC scale Crying Duration	The breastfeeding was determined to be more effective than the sucrose and control groups.
Zurita Cruz et al., 2017	Vaccination	A controlled, single-blind phase III clinical trial	Breastfeeding, milk substitutes (MS) and without applying any analgesic application (control).	Crying duration and pediatric pain scale	It was found that breastfeeding was effective in management of acute pain by vaccination in infants younger than six months than milk substitute and control groups
Fallah et al., 2017	Vaccination 120 healthy term infants	Randomized trial	Breastfeeding group Kangaroo mother care (KMC) Swaddling	Pain score	Breastfeeding was more effective than KMC and swaddling in order to reduce BCG vaccination pain in healthy term infants.
Erkul & Efe, 2017	Vaccination 100 infants	Randomized controlled experimental trial	Breastfeeding group Control group	NIPS score	Breastfeeding prevented increased heart rates, duration of crying, NIPS, decreasing oxygen saturation and reduced pain during the invasive procedures in newborns more compared to control group.
Hashemi et al., 2016	Vaccination 131 healthy term infants	Randomized double-blind intervention	Swaddled group Breastfed group combined group (Breastfed + Swaddled) Control group	Neonatal Facial Coding System (NFCS) Physiological responses	There was a statistically significant difference in mean pain level in the three intervention groups compared to the control group
Chiabi et al., 2016	Heel lance 100 infants	Randomized clinical trials	Breastfeeding group 30% glucose group	Neonatal Infant Pain Scale.	Breastfeeding had a higher analgesic effect compared to 30% glucose solution.

Table 4. (Continued)

Authors	Procedure	Method	Groups	Measurement	Results
Zhu et al., 2015	Heel lance, 250 healthy-term infants	Randomized controlled trial	Breastfeeding (BF), music therapy (MT) and combined breastfeeding and music therapy (BF+MT)	Neonatal Infant Pain Scale (NIPS), latency to first cry and duration of first crying.	BF could significantly reduce pain response in healthy-term infants during heel lancing. MT did not increase the pain relief effect of BF.
Esfahani et al., 2013	Vaccination 96 infants	Randomized controlled trial	Breast feeding group Massage group Control groups	NIPS	In vaccination, breastfeeding had a more analgesic effect compared to massage therapy.
Marin Gabriel et al., 2013	Heel lance One hundred thirty-six healthy term infants.	Randomized controlled trial	Group breastfeeding with skin-to-skin contact (SSC) (n = 35); Group sucrose with SSC (n = 35); SSC Group (n = 33); or Sucrose Group (n = 33)	NIPS	This study revealed that BF plus SSC provided the highest analgesia in healthy term infants during heel lance procedure compared to other kinds of non-pharmacological analgesia.
Boroumandfar et al., 2013	Vaccination 144 infants	Randomized controlled trial	Breastfeeding, Apocopate spray, Control group	NIPS	In vaccination, breastfeeding had a more analgesic effect, than vapocoolant spray applied before vaccination.
Gupta et al., 2013	Vaccination 90 infants	Randomized, placebo-controlled trial	EMLA cream with breastfeeding EMLA cream with oral distilled water Placebo cream with oral distilled water	Duration of crying, latency of onset of cry and Modified Facial Coding Score	During vaccination, topical EMLA effectively relieved pain and had a synergistic effect in analgesia in combination with breastfeeding in infants.

Authors	Procedure	Method	Groups	Measurement	Results
Goswami et al., 2013	Vaccination 120 infants	Randomized, placebo controlled trial	Breast feed group, 25% dextrose fed group Distilled water fed group	Duration of crying after vaccination Modified Facial Coding Score (MFCS)	Direct breastfeeding and 25% dextrose had an analgesic effect in young infants vaccinated with DPT in infants under 3 months of age.
Holsti, Oberlander & Brant, 2011	Blood collection 57 infants	Randomized, controlled trial	BF group, Soother group	The Behavioral Indicators of Infant Pain (BIIP)	Breastfeeding did not relieve pain during blood collection.
Okan et al., 2010	Heel lance 107 neonates	Randomized, controlled trial	Breastfed with skin-to-skin contact (group 1, n = 35) Skin-to-skin contact but no breastfeeding (group 2, n = 36) lying on the table before, during, and after painful stimulus (group 3, n = 36)	Heart rate and oxygen saturation changes, Duration of crying and grimacing.	In healthy term infants, the skin-to-skin contact with the mother and the breastfeeding with skin-to-skin contact decreased both physiological and behavioral pain response.
Abdel Razek & El-Dein, 2009	Vaccination 120 infants	Quasi-experimental design	Breastfeeding + skin to skin contact group Control group	Facial Pain Rating Scale and Neonatal/Infant Pain Scale (NIPS)	Breast-feeding and skin-to-skin contact led crying to be significantly lower in immunized infants.

Table 5. The results of the studies using expressed breast milk during painful procedures

Authors	Procedure	Method	Groups	Measurement	Results
Peng et al., 2018	Heel lance procedures. 109 preterm infants	A prospective, randomized controlled trial	Sucking+ breast milk Sucking+breast milk+tucking Routine care	PIPP	Using sucking+breast milk +tucking and sucking+breast milk together effectively decreased preterm infants' mild and moderate-to-severe pain during heel lance procedures.
Hsieh et al., 2018	Heel Lance 20 preterm infants	Prospective study	Breast Milk, 10% dextrose water, Distilled water (placebo) Control group	PIPP	Significant differences were found between BM/control group. Breast Milk decreased pain.
Hatami Bavarsad et al., 2018	Vaccination 100 infants	Randomized controlled trial	Control group (no feeding); the Breastfed group; the bottle-fed Mother's milk group Powdered formula group	DAN	Breastfeeding decreased pain level in infants during painful procedures.
Bozlak & Dolgun, 2018	Retinopathy of prematurity 87 premature infants	Randomized controlled trial	Swaddling with oral administration of sucrose Swaddling with oral administration of breast milk Swaddling with oral administration of distilled water (control)	PIPP	There was no significant difference among three groups in terms of Premature Infant Pain Profile scores.

Authors	Procedure	Method	Groups	Measurement	Results
Desai et al., 2017	Suctioning 108 infants	Randomized controlled clinical trial	Expressed Breast Milk (EBM) Swaddling Sucrose	PIPP	Difference was not found among EBM, swaddling and sucrose in relieving suction-related pain.
Şener Taplak & Erdem, 2017	Retinopathy of prematurity (ROP) examination. 60 preterm infants	Double-blind randomized controlled experimental study	Breast milk group, Sucrose group Control/distilled water group	PIPP	The values of the preterm infants in the breast milk group returned to baseline values more quickly after the ROP examination and these infants recovered faster compared to those in the sucrose group
Simonse, Mulder & van Beek, 2012	Heel Lance 71 infants	Randomized controlled clinical trial	Breast milk group, Sucrose group	PIPP	Any significant difference was not found between breast milk and sucrose groups in terms of PIPP mean scores
Bueno et al., 2012	Heel Lance 113 infants	A noninferiority randomized controlled trial	25% glucose group Expressed breast milk	PIPP Crying duration	PIPP scores and crying time had a lower impact on EBM than 25% glucose during heel lance procedure.
Ozdoğan et al., 2010	Heel Lance 142 infants		Single-dose breast milk Single-dose sterile water Single-dose 12.5% sucrose Two-dose breast milk Two-dose sterile water Two-dose 12.5% sucrose	Crying duration Neonatal facial coding system	Single or double-dose breast milk did not have any effect on relieving pain in infants.

Table 6. The results of the studies using expressed breast milk smell during painful procedures

Authors	Procedure	Method	Groups	Measurement	Results
Baudesson de Chanville et al., 2017	Venipuncture	Randomized controlled clinical trial	Maternal milk smell group; Control group	PIPP	Median PIPP score was significantly lower during venipuncture in infants in maternal milk smell group than the control group
Küçük Alemdar and Kardaş Özdemir, 2017	Peripheral cannulation 136 preterm infants	Randomized controlled trial	Breast milk smell group; Maternal voice group	PIPP	There was no difference between the groups before the peripheral cannulation procedure in terms of the total Premature Infant Pain Profile (PIPP) scores
Neshat et al., 2017	Bloodletting 135 preterm infants	Randomized controlled trial	Vanilla smell group; Breast milk smell group; Control Group	Heart rate; Blood oxygen saturation	Breast milk smell affected significantly the changes of neonatal heart rate and blood oxygen saturation during and after venipuncture and reduced the variability of premature infants' heart rate and blood oxygen saturation
Badiee, Asghari & Mohammadizadeh, 2017	Heel Lance 50 preterm infants	Randomized controlled trial	Breast milk smell; Formula milk smell	PIPP; Period of crying and salivary cortisol before and after heel lancing	Breast milk smell has an analgesic effect in preterm infants.
Akcan and Polat, 2016	Heel Lance 102 newborn infants	Randomized controlled trial	Breast milk smell group; Amniotic fluid smell group; Lavender smell group; Control Group	NIPS; Heart rate; Oxygen saturation	The smells of lavender and breast milk prevent the increased heart rates, NIPS, decreasing oxygen saturation and alleviated pain in newborns during the invasive procedures more compared to amniotic fluid or control group
Jebreili et al., 2015	Venipuncture 135 preterm infants	Randomized controlled trial	Breast milk smell group; Vanilla smell group; Control Group	PIPP	Breastmilk smell has a more calming effect on premature infants than vanilla smell.

In their study, Rattaz et al., determined that breast milk smell and vanilla smell reduced grimacing of newborns during heel lance procedure and breast milk smell alone was effective on reducing the stress of newborns after venipuncture procedure (Rattaz et al., 2005).

CONCLUSION

Numerous painful interventions are applied to newborns and infants. In this study, we evaluated the findings of studies including breast milk alone, breast milk odor and breastfeeding in reducing pain related to interventions. The results obtained from the studies showed that breastfeeding was more effective on reducing pain during painful interventions such as heel lance, aspiration and vaccination in newborns and infants, compared to studies using breast milk or breast milk smell alone. It can be asserted that breastfeeding shows this effect since it is composed of analgesic effect of breast milk, skin-to-skin contact and mother's smell. According to these results, it is recommended that breastfeeding be used as a non-pharmacological method during painful interventions in newborns and infants, and further studies on breast milk and breast milk smell are recommended.

REFERENCES

Abdel Razek, A., Az El-Dein, N. (2009). Effect of breast-feeding on pain relief during infant immunization injections. *Int J Nurs Pract*, 15(2):99-104. doi: 10.1111/j.1440-172X.2009.01728.x.

Akcan, E., Polat, S. (2016). Comparative effect of the smells of amniotic fluid, breast milk, and lavender on newborns' pain during heel lance. *Breastfeed Med*, 11: 309-314.

Akcan, E., Polat, S. (2017). Pain in newborns and the nurse's role in pain management. *ACU Health Science Journal,* (2):64-69 (in Turkish).

Aliefendioğlu, D., Güzoğlu, N. (2015). Pain in Neonatale. *Journal of Child Health and Disease,* 58:35-42.(in Turkish).

Altun, O., Ozek, E. (2005). Analgesic effect of expressed breast milk: lactose or fat content--which one is important? *Acta Paediatr,* 94(7):980.

Altun-Koroglu, O., Ozek, E., Bilgen, H., Cebeci, D. (2010). Hindmilk for procedural pain in term neonates. *Turk J Pediatr,* 52(6):623-629.

American Academy of Pediatrics Committee on Fetus and Newborn and Section on Anesthesiology and Pain Medicine. (2016). Prevention and management of procedural pain in the neonate: an update. *Pediatrics,* 137(2):1–13. doi:10.1542/peds.2015-4271.

Anand KJS. (2017). Defining pain in newborns: need for a uniform taxonomy? *Acta Paediatr,* 106(9):1438-1444. doi: 10.1111/apa.13936.

Anand, K. J., Garg, S., Rovnaghi, C. R., et al. (2007). Ketamine reduces the cell death following inflammatory pain in newborn rat brain. *Pediatr Res,* 62:283-290.

Aoyama, S., Toshima, T., Saito, Y., Konishi, N., Motoshige, K., Ishikawa, N., Nakamura, K., Kobayashi, M. (2010). Maternal breast milk odour induces frontal lobe activation in neonates: A NIRS study. *Early Hum Dev,* 86: 541-545.

Badiee Z, Asghari M, Mohammadizadeh M. (2013). The calming effect of maternal breast milk odor on premature infants. *Pediatr Neonatol,*54:322-325.

Ballweg, D. (2007). Neonatal and Pediatric Pain Management: Standards and Application. *Paediatrics and Child Health,*17:61-66.

Barker, D. P., Rutter, N. (1995). Exposure to invasive procedures in neonatal intensive care unit admissions. *Arch Dis Child Fetal Neonatal Ed*, 72:47-48.

Barrett, T., Kent, S., Voudouris, N. (2000). Does melatonin modulate beta-endorphin, corticosterone, and pain threshold? *Life Sci,* 66(6):467-76.

Baudesson de Chanville, A., Brevaut-Malaty, V., Garbi, A., Tosello, B., Baumstarck, K., Gire, C. (2017). Analgesic effect of maternal human milk odor on premature neonates: A randomized controlled trial. *J Hum Lact,* 33(2):300-308. doi: 10.1177/0890334417693225.

Bellieni, C. V., Tei, M., Cornacchione, S., et al. (2017). Pain perception in NICU: A pilot questionnaire. *J Matern Fetal Neonatal Med.*, 17:1-8.

Beltramini, A., Milojevic, K., Pateron, D. (2017). Pain assessment in newborns, infants, and children. Pediatr Ann, 1;46(10):e387-e395. doi: 10.3928/19382359-20170921-03.

Blass, E. M. (1997). Milk-induced hypoalgesia in human newborns. *Pediatrics,* 99(6):825-829.

Blass, E. M., Fitzgerald, E. (1988). Milk-induced analgesia and comforting in 10-day-old rats: opioid mediation. *Pharmacol Biochem Behav,* 29(1):9-13.

Blass, E. M., Miller, L. W. (2001). Effects of colostrum in newborn humans: dissociation between analgesic and cardiac effects. *J Dev Behav Pediatr,* 22(6):385–390. doi:10.1097/ 00004703-200112000-00006.

Blount, R. L., Loiselle, K. A. (2009). Behavioural assessment of pediatric pain. *Pain Res Manage*, 14:47-52.

Boroumandfar, K., Khodaei, F., Abdeyazdan, Z., Maroufi, M. (2013). Comparison of vaccination-related pain in infants who receive vapocoolant spray and breastfeeding during injection. *Iran J Nurs Midwifery Res,* 18(1):33-7.

Bozlak, Ş., Dolgun, G. (2017). Effect of nonpharmacologic pain control during examination for retinopathy of prematurity. *J Obstet Gynecol Neonatal Nurs,* 46(5):709-715. doi: 10.1016/j.jogn.2017.06.008.

Brand, K., Canchi, N. (2013). Pain assessment in children. *Anaesthesia & Intensive Care Medicine,* 14:228-231.

Britto, C. D., Rao, Pn S., Nesargi, S., Nair, S., Rao, S., Thilagavathy, T., Ramesh, A., Bhat, S. (2014). PAIN perception and assessment of painful procedures in the NICU. *J Trop Pediatr,* 60(6):422-7. doi: 10.1093/tropej/fmu039.

Brummelte, S., Grunau, R. E., Chau, V., et al. (2012). Procedural pain and brain development in premature newborns. *Ann Neurol,* 71: 385-396.

Bucher, H. U., Baumgartner, R., Bucher, N., Seiler, M., Fauchere, J. C. (2000). Artificial sweetener reduces nociceptive reaction in term newborn infants. *Early Hum Dev,* 59(1):51–60.

Bueno, M., Stevens, B., de Camargo, P. P., Toma, E., Krebs, V. L., Kimura, A. F. (2012). Breast milk and glucose for pain relief in preterm infants: a noninferiority randomized controlled trial. *Pediatrics,* 129(4):664-670

Buntinx, M., Moreels, M., Vandenabeele, F., Lambrichts, I., Raus, J., Steels, P., Stinissen, P., Ameloot, M. (2004). Cytokine-induced cell death in human oligodendroglial cell lines: I. Synergistic effects of IFN-gamma and TNF-alpha on apoptosis. *J Neurosci Res,* 15;76(6):834-45.

Carbajal, R., Rousset, A., Danan, C., et al. (2008). Epidemiology and treatment of painful procedures in neonates in intensive care units. *JAMA,* 300(1):60–70pmid:18594041.

Chiabi, A., Eloundou, E., Mah, E., Nguefack, S., Mekone, I., Mbonda, E. (2016). Evaluation of breast-feeding and 30% glucose solution as analgesic measures in indigenous African term neonates. *J Clin Neonatol,*5(1):46–50. doi:10.4103/2249-4847.173269.

Cignaccoa, E., Hamersb, J., Lingenc, A., et al. (2009). Neonatal procedural pain exposure and pain management in ventilated preterm infants during the first 14 days of life. *Swıss Med Wkly,* 139:226-232.

Codipietro, L., Ceccarelli, M., Ponzone, A. (2008). A randomized, controlled trial breastfeeding or oral sucrose solution in term neonates receiving heel lance. *Pediatrics,* 122(3): 716-721.

Cruz, M. D., Fernandes, A. M., Oliveira, C. R. (2016). Epidemiology of painful procedures performed in neonates: systematic review of observational studies. *Eur J Pain,* 20(4):489-98. doi: 10.1002/ejp.757.

Çöçelli, L. P., Bacaksız, B. D., Ovayolu, N. (2008). The role of the nurse in the treatment of pain. *Gaziantep Medical Journal,14*:53-58. (in Turkish).

Derebent, E., Yiğit, R. (2006). Pain and Management in Newborn. *Cumhuriyet University School of Nursing Journal,*10(2): 42-49.

Desai, S., Nanavati, R. N., Nathani, R., Kabra, N. (2017). Effect of Expressed breast milk versus swaddling versus oral sucroseadministration on pain associated with suctioning in preterm neonates on assisted ventilation: A Randomized Controlled Trial. *Indian J Palliat Care,* 23(4):372-378. doi: 10.4103/IJPC.IJPC_84_17.

Diego, M. A., Field, T., Reif, M. H. (2009). Procedural Pain Heart Rate Responses in Massaged Preterm Infants. *Infant Behav Dev.,*32:226-229.

Dikmen, Y. (2012). Mechanical Ventilation. Basics of clinical practice. Güneş Medical Bookstores, İstanbul,171-185.

Dilli, D., Küçük, I. G., Dallar, Y. (2009). Interventions to reduce pain during vaccination in infancy. *Journal of Pediatric,* 154 (3): 385-390.

Dunwoody, C. J., Krenzischek, D. A., Pasero, C., Rathmell, J. P., Polomano, R. C. (2008). Assessment, physiological monitoring, and consequences of inadequately treated acute pain. *J Perianesth Nurs,*23:15-27.

Efe, E., Ozer, Z. C. (2007). The use of breast-feeding for pain relief during neonatal immunization injections. *Appl Nurs Res,*20(1):10–16. doi:10.1016/j.apnr.2005.10.005.

Erdine, S. (2007). Pain Mechanisms and General Approach to Pain. In: Erdine S: *Pain* (3rd Edition). Nobel Medical Bookstores, Istanbul, 37-49.

Erkul, M., Efe, E. (2017). Efficacy of breastfeeding on babies' pain during vaccinations. *Breastfeed Med,* 12:110-115. doi: 10.1089/bfm. 2016.0141.

Esfahani, M. S., Sheykhi, S., Abdeyazdan, Z., Jodakee, M., Boroumandfar, K. (2013). A comparative study on vaccination pain inthe methods of massage therapy and mothers' breast feeding during injection of infants referring to Navabsafavi HealthCare Center in Isfahan. *Iran J Nurs Midwifery Res,* 18(6):494-8.

Fallah, R., Naserzadeh, N., Ferdosian, F., Binesh, F. (2017). Comparison of effect of kangaroo mother care, breastfeeding and swaddling on Bacillus Calmette-Guerin vaccination pain score in healthy term neonates by a clinical trial. *J Matern Fetal Neonatal Med,* 30(10):1147-1150. doi: 10.1080/14767058.2016.1205030.

Fitzgerald, M., Walker, S. (2006). Infant pain traces. *Pain,* 5;125(3):204-5.

Gad, R. F., Dowling, D. A., Abusaad, F. E., Bassiouny, M. R., Abd El Aziz, M. A. (2019). Oral sucrose versus breastfeeding in managing infants' ımmunization-related pain: A randomized controlled trial. *MCN Am J Matern Child Nurs*, 44(2):108-114.

Gibbins, S., Stevens, B. (2001). Mechanisms of sucrose and non-nutritive sucking in procedural pain management in infants. *Pain Res Manag,* 6(1):21-8.

Goswami, G., Upadhyay, A., Gupta, N. K., Chaudhry, R., Chawla, D., Sreenivas, V. (2013). Comparison of analgesic effect of direct breastfeeding, oral 25% dextrose solution and placebo during 1st DPT vaccination in healthy term infants: A randomized, placebo controlled trial. *Indian Pediatr,* 50(7):649-53.

Gradin, M., Finnstrom, O., Schollin, J. (2004). Feeding and oral glucose—additive effects on pain reduction in newborns. *Early Hum Dev,* 77(1–2):57–65. doi:10.1016/j.earlhumdev.2004.01.003.

Gray, L., Miller, L. W., Philipp, B. L., Blass, E. M. (2002). Breastfeeding ıs analgesic in healthy newborns. *Pediatrics,* 109(4):590-593. doi:10.1177/08934402018003015.

Grunau, R. E. (2013). Neonatal pain in very preterm infants: Long-term effects on brain, neurodevelopment and pain reactivity. *Rambam Maimonides Medical Journal,* 4(4), e0025.

Grunau, R. E. (2013). Neonatal pain in very preterm ınfants: Long-term effects on brain, neurodevelopment and pain reactivity. *Rambam Maimonides Med J,* 4:1-13.

Grunau, R. E., Weinberg, J., Whitfield, M. F. (2004). Neonatal procedural pain and preterm infant cortisol response to novelty at 8 month. *Pediatrics,* 114:78-84.

Gupta, N. K., Upadhyay, A., Agarwal, A., Goswami, G., Kumar, J., Sreenivas, V. (2013). Randomized controlled trial of topical EMLA and breastfeeding for reducing pain during wDPT vaccination. *Eur J Pediatr,* 172(11):1527-33. doi: 10.1007/s00431-013-2076-6.

Hansson, E. (2006). Could chronic pain and spread of pain sensation be induced and maintained by glial activation? *Acta Physiol,* 187:321-327.

Hashemi, F., Taheri, L., Ghodsbin, F., Pishva, N., Vossoughi, M. (2016). Comparing the effect of swaddling and breastfeeding and their combined effect on the pain induced by BCG vaccination in infants referring to Motahari Hospital, Jahrom, 2010-2011. *Appl Nurs Res*, 29:217-21. doi: 10.1016/j.apnr.2015.05.013.

Hatami Bavarsad, Z., Hemati, K., Sayehmiri, K., Asadollahi, P., Abangah, G., Azizi, M., Asadollahi, K. (2018). Effects of breast milk on pain severity during muscular injection of hepatitis B vaccine in neonates in a teaching hospital in Iran. *Arch Pediatr*, 25(6):365-370. doi: 10.1016/j.arcped.2018.06.001.

Henry, P. R., Haubold, K., Dobrzykowski, T. M. (2004). Pain in the healthy full-term neonate: Efficacy and safety of interventions. *Newborn and Infant Nursing Reviews*,4:106-113.

Holsti, L., Oberlander, T. F., Brant, R. (2011). Does breastfeeding reduce acute procedural pain in preterm infants in the neonatal intensive care unit? A Randomized Clinical Trial. *Pain*, 152 (11): 2575–2581. doi: 10.1016/j.pain.2011.07.022.

Hsieh, K. H., Chen, S. J., Tsao, P. C., Wang, C. C., Huang, C. F., Lin, C. M., Chou, Y. L., Chen, W. Y., Chan, I. C. (2018). The analgesic effect of non-pharmacological interventions to reduce procedural pain in preterm neonates. *Pediatr Neonatol*, 59(1):71-76. doi: 10.1016/j.pedneo.2017.02.001.

Jatana, S. K., Dalal, S. S., Wilson, C. G. (2003). Analgesic effect of oral glucose in neonates. *Med J Armed Forces India*, 59(2):100–104.

Jebreili, M., Neshat, H., Seyyedrasouli, A., Ghojazade, M., Hosseini, M. B., Hamishehkar, H. (2015). Comparison of breastmilk odor and vanilla odor on mitigating premature infants' response to pain during and after venipuncture. *Breastfeed Med*, 10(7):362-5. doi: 10.1089/bfm.2015.0060.

Johnston, C., Barrington, K. J., Taddio, A., Carbajal, R., Filion, F. (2011). Pain in Canadian NICUs have we improved over the past 12 years? *Clin J Pain*, 27:225-232.

Johnston, C. C., Collinge, J. M., Henderson, S. J., Anand, K. J. (1997). A cross-sectional survey of pain and pharmacological analgesia in Canadian neonatal intensive care units. *Clin J Pain,* 13:308.

Krishnan, L. (2013). Pain relief in neonates. *Journal of Neonatal Surgery,* 2(2):19.

Küçükoğlu Alemdar, D., Kardaş Özdemir, F. (2017). Effects of having preterm infants smell amniotic fluid, mother's milk, and mother's odor during heel stick procedure on pain, physiological parameters, and crying duration. *Breastfeed Med*, 17. doi: 10.1089/bfm.2017.0006.

Lago, P., Guadagni, A., Merazzi, D., et al. (2005). Pain management in the neonatal intensive care unit: A national survey in Italy. *Paediatr Anaesth,* 15:925-31.

Marín Gabriel, M. Á., del Rey Hurtado de Mendoza, B., Jiménez Figueroa, L., Medina, V., Iglesias Fernández, B., Vázquez Rodríguez, M., Escudero Huedo, V., Medina Malagón, L. (2013). Analgesia with breastfeeding in addition to skin-to-skin contact during heel prick. *Arch Dis Child Fetal Neonatal Ed,* 98(6):F499-503. doi: 10.1136/archdischild-2012-302921.

Mathai, S., Natrajan, N., Rajalakshmi, N. R. (2006). A comparative study of non-pharmacological methods to reduce pain in neonates. *Indian Pediatr,* 43:1070–1075.

Maxwell, L. G., Malavolta, C. P., Fraga, M. V. Assessment of pain in the neonate. Clin Perinatol. 2013 Sep;40(3):457-69. doi: 10.1016/j.clp.2013.05.001.

Morais, A. P. S., Façanha, S. M. A., Rabelo, S. N., Silva, A. V. S., Queiroz, M. V. O., & Chaves, E. M. C. (2016). Non-pharmacological measures in the pain management in newborns: Nursing care. Revista Rene, 17(3), 435e442.

Moultrie, F., Slater, R., Hartley, C. (2017). Improving the treatment of infant pain. *Current Opinion in Supportive and Palliative Care,* 11(2), 112–117. http://doi:10.1097/SPC.0000000000000270.

Neshat, H., Jebreili, M., Seyyedrasouli, A., et al. (2016). Effects of breast milk and vanilla odors on premature neonate's heart rate and blood oxygen saturation during and after venipuncture. *Pediatr Neonatol,* 57:225-231.

Nishitani, S., Miyamura, T., Tagawa, M., et al. (2009). The calming effect of a maternal breast milk odor on the human newborn infant. *Neurosci Res,* 63:66-71.

Noel, M., Chambers, C. T., McGrath, P. J., Klein, R. M., Stewart, S. H. (2012). The influence of children's pain memories on subsequent pain experience. *Pain,* 153(8):1563-72. doi: 10.1016/j.pain.2012.02.020.

Okan, F., Ozdil, A., Bulbul, A., Yapici, Z., Nuhoglu, A. (2010). Analgesic effects of skin to skin contact and breast-feeding in procedural pain in healthy term neonates. *Ann Trop Paediatr,* 30(2):119–128. doi:10.1179/146532810× 12703902516121.

Okan, F., Ozdil, A., Bulbul, A., Yapici, Z., Nuhoglu, A. (2010). Analgesic effects of skin-to-skin contact and breastfeeding in procedural pain in healthy term neonates. *Ann Trop Paediatr, 30*(2):119-28. doi: 10.1179/146532810X12703902516121.

Ors, R., Ozek, E., Baysoy, G., Cebeci, D., Bilgen, H., Turkuner, M., et al. (1999). Comparison of sucrose and human milk on pain response in newborns. *Eur J Pediatr,* 158(1):63-66.

Ou-Yang, M. C., Chen, I. L., Chen, C. C., Chung, M. Y., Chen, F. S., Huang, H. C. (2013). Expressed breast milk for procedural pain in preterm neonates: A randomized, double-blind, placebo-controlled trial. *Acta Paediatr,* 102(1):15- 21.

Ozdogan, T., Akman, I., Cebeci, D., Bilgen, H., Ozek, E. (2010). Comparison of two doses of breast milk and sucrose during neonatal heel prick. *Pediatr Int,* 52(2):175–179. doi:10.1111/j .1442-200X.2009.02921.x.

Padhye, N. S., Williams, A. L., Khattak, A. Z., Lasky, R. E. (2009). Heart rate variability in response to pain stimulus in VLBW. Infants Followed Longitudinally During NICU Stay. *Dev Psychobiol*, 51: 638-649.

Peng, H. F., Yin, T., Yang, L., Wang, C., Chang, Y. C., Jeng, M. J., Liaw, J. J. (2018). Non-nutritive sucking, oral breast milk, and facilitated tucking relieve preterm infant pain during heel-stick procedures: A prospective, randomized controlled trial. *Int J Nurs Stud,*77:162-170. doi: 10.1016/j.ijnurstu.2017.10.001.

Perrone, S., Bellieni, C. V., Negro, S., et al. (2017). Oxidative stress as a physiological pain response in full-term newborns. *Oxid Med Cell Longev*, 2017:3759287:1-7.

Phillips, R. M., Chantry, C. J., Galagher, M. P. (2005). Analgesic effect of breastfeeding or pacifier use with maternal holding in term infants. *Ambul Pediatr,* 5(6): 359-364.

Ranger, M., Chau, C. M. Y., Garg, A., et al. (2013). Neonatal pain-related stress predicts cortical thickness at age 7 years in children born very preterm. *PLoS ONE,* 8:e76702.

Rattaz, C., Goubet, N., Bullinger, A. (2005). The calming effect of a familiar odor on fullterm newborns. *J Dev Behav Pediatr,* 26:86-92

Reece-Stremtan, S., Gray, L. (2016). ABM Clinical Protocol #23: Nonpharmacological Management of Procedure-Related Pain in the Breastfeeding Infant, Revised 2016. *Breastfeed Med,* 11:425-429.

Roofthooft, D. W., Simons, S. H., Anand, K. J., Tibboel D., Dick, M. V. (2014). Eight years later, are we still hurting newborn infants? *Neonatology,* 105:218.

Rosali, L., Nesargi, S., Mathew, S., Vasu, U., Rao, S. P., Bhat, S. (2015). Efficacy of expressed breast milk in reducing pain during ROP screening--A randomized controlled trial. *J Trop Pediatr,* 61(2):135-8.

Sahoo, J. P., Rao, S., Nesargi, S., Ranjit, T., Ashok, C., Bhat, S. (2013). Expressed breast milk vs 25% dextrose in procedural pain in neonates, a double blind randomized controlled trial. *Indian Pediatr,* 50(2):203-207.

Shah PS, Herbozo C, Aliwalas LL, Shah VS. (2012). Breastfeeding or breast milk for procedural pain in neonates. *Cochrane Database Syst Rev,* 12;12:CD004950.

Simons, S. H., van Dijk, M., Anand, K. S., et al. (2003). Do we still hurt newborn babies? A prospective study of procedural pain and analgesia in neonates. *Arch Pediatr Adolesc Med,*157:1058-1064.

Simonse, E., Mulder, P. G., van Beek, R. H. (2012). Analgesic effect of breast milk versus sucrose for analgesia during heel lance in late preterm infants. *Pediatrics,* 129(4):657-63. doi: 10.1542/peds.2011-2173.

Skogsdal, Y., Eriksson, M., Schollin, J. (1997). Analgesia in newborns given oral glucose. *Acta Paediatr,* 86(2):217–220. 55.

Slater, L., Asmerom, Y., Boskovic, D. S., Bahjri, K., Plank, M. S., Angeles, K. R., Phillips, R., Deming, D., Ashwal, S., Hougland, K., Fayard, E., Angeles, D. M. (2012). Procedural pain and oxidative stress in premature neonates. *J Pain,* 13(6):590-97.

Slater, R., Fabrizi, L., Worley, A., et al. (2010). Premature infants display increased noxious-evoked neuronal activity in the brain compared to healthy age-matched term-born infants. *NeuroImage,* 52:583-589.

Standley, J. M., & Swedberg, O. (2011). NICU music therapy: Post hoc analysis of an early intervention clinical program. *The Arts in Psychotherapy,* 38(1), 36e40.

Stevens, B., Johnston, C., Taddio, A., Gibbins S, Yamada J. (2014). The premature infant pain profile-revised (PIPP-R): İnitial validation and feasibility. *Clin J Pain,* 30:238.

Stevens, B., McGrath, P., Gibbins, S., et al. (2003). Procedural pain in newborns at risk for neurologic impairment. *Pain,* 105:27-35.

Stevens, B. J., Gibbins, S., Yamada, J., et al. (2014). The premature infant pain profile-revised (PIPP-R): Initial validation and feasibility. *Clin J Pain,* 30:238-43.

Şener Taplak, A., Erdem E. (2017). A Comparison of Breast Milk and Sucrose in Reducing Neonatal Pain During Eye Exam for Retinopathy of Prematurity. *Breastfeed Med,* 12:305-310. doi: 10.1089/bfm.2016.0122.

Talos, D. M., Follett PL, Folkerth RD, et al. (2006). Developmental regulation of AMPA receptor subunit expression in forebrain and relationship to regional susceptibility to hypoxic/ischemic injury: Part II. Human cerebral white matter and cortex. Steward O, ed. *The Journal of Comparative Neurology,* 497(1):61-77.

Tekgündüz, K. Ş., Polat, S., Gürol, A., Apay Ejder, S. (2019). Oral glucose and listening to lullaby to decrease pain in preterm infants supported with NCPAP: A Randomized Controlled Trial. *Pain Management Nursing,* 20;54-61, doi:org/10.1016/j.pmn.2018.04.008.

Törüner, E., Büyükgönenç, L. (2011). Basic Nursing Approaches to Child Health. Göktuğ Publishing: Ankara,146-170. (in Turkish).

Uğurlu, E. S. (2017). Non-pharmacological pain relief methods of invasive procedures in children. *ACU Health Science Journal,*(4):198-201. (in Turkish).

Upadhyay, A., Aggarwal, R., Narayan, S., Joshi, M., Paul, V. K., Deorari, A. K. (2004). Analgesic effect of expressed breast milk in procedural pain in term neonates: a randomized, placebo controlled, double-blind trial. *Acta Paediatr,* 93(4): 518–522. doi:10.1080/0803 5250410022792.

Uyan, Z. S., Ozek, E., Bilgen, H., Cebeci, D., Akman, I. (2005). Effect of foremilk and hindmilk on simple procedural pain in newborns. *Pediatr Int,* 47(3):252–257. doi:10.1111/j.1442- 200x.2005.02055.x.

Vinall, J., Grunau, R.E. (2014). Impact of repeated procedural pain-related stress in infants born very preterm. *Pediatr Res,* 75:584-587.

Walker, S. M. Neonatal pain. *Paediatr Anaesth.* 2014 Jan;24(1):39-48. doi: 10.1111/pan.12293.

Walter-Nicolet, E., Annequin, D., Biran, V., Mitanchez, D., Tourniaire, B. (2010). Pain management in newborns. *Pediatr Drugs,* 12(6): 354-364.

Weissman, A., Aranovitch, M., Blazer, S., Zimmer, E. Z. (2009). Heellancing in newborns: Behavioral and spectral analysis assessment of pain control methods. *Pediatrics,*124(5): e921–e926. doi:10.1542/peds.2009-0598.

Williams, A. L., Khattak, A. Z., Garza, C. N., Lasky, R. E. (2009). The behavioral pain response to heelstick in preterm neonates studied longitudinally: Description, development, determinants and components. *Early Hum Dev,* 85:369-374.

Witt, N., Coynor, S., Edwards, C., & Bradshaw, H. (2016). A guide to pain assessment and management in the neonate. Current Emergency and Hospital Medicine Reports, 4(1), 1e10.

Witt, N., Coynor, S., Edwards, C., Bradshaw, H. (2016). A guide to pain assessment and management in the neonate. *Current Emergency and*

Hospital Medicine Reports, 4, 1–10. http://doi:10.1007/s40138-016-0089-y.

Yiğit, Ş., Ecevit, A., Altun Köroğlu, Ö. (2015). Pain and Treatment Guide in Newborn Period 2015. Türk Neonatoloji Association.

Yiğit, Ş., Ecevit, A., Altun Köroğlu, Ö. (2018). Turkish Neonatal Society guideline on the neonatal pain and its management. *Turk Pediatri Ars,* 53(Suppl 1): S161-S171 (in Turkish).

Yilmaz, F., Arikan, D. (2011). The effects of various interventions to newborns on pain and duration of crying. *J Clin Nurs,* 20(7–8):1008–1017. doi:10.1111/j.1365- 2702.2010.03356.x.

Young, K. D. (2005). Pediatric procedural pain. Annals of Emergency Medicine, 45(2), 160e171.

Zahr, L. K., Balian, S. (1995). Responses of premature infants to routine nursing interventions and noise in the NICU. *Nurs Res,* 44:179-185.

Zempsky, W. T., Schechter, N. L. (2003). What's new in the management of pain in children. *Pediatrics,* 24:337-347.

Zhu, J., Hong-Gu, H., Zhou, X., Wei, H., Gao, Y., Ye, B., Liu, Z., Chan, S. W. (2015). Pain relief effect of breast feeding and music therapy during heel lance for healthy-term neonates in China: A randomized controlled trial. Midwifery, 31:365–372. doi: 10.1016/j.midw.2014.11.001.

Zurita-Cruz, J. N., Rivas-Ruiz, R., Gordillo-Álvarez, V., Villasis-Keever, M. Á. (2017). Breastfeeding for acute pain control on infants: A randomized controlled trial. Nutr Hosp., 30;34(2):301-307. doi: 10.20960/nh.163.

BIOGRAPHICAL SKETCHES

Sevinç POLAT, PhD

Affiliation: Prof. PhD, RN. Department of Pediatric Nursing, Yozgat Bozok University, Yozgat, Turkey

Business Address: Yozgat Bozok University

Research and Professional Experience: Child Health and Disease Nursing

Honors:
1- Şener Taplak A, Parlak Gürol A, Polat S, Polat M F. Forensic Cases Related to Children Reflected in the Media. International II. *Forensic Nursing and I.* Social Work Congress. 3-4 November 2016. Kırıkkale (Oral Presentation Award).
2- Polat S, Duzgun M. V, Polat M. F, Gurol A. The views of nursing students about participating in scientific activities. *Symposium on Professionalization Process in Student Nurses*. 30-31 March 2016. Yozgat (Oral Presentation First Prize).
3- Polat S, Yalman E, Acarbas F, Akturan E. Problems of Nursing Education from the Eyes of Academicians: Qualitative Study. Symposium on the Process of Professionalization in Student Nurses, 30-31 March 2016, Yozgat (Verbal Paper Second Prize).
4- Polat S, Sener Taplak A, Daar G, Yuzer S. *Mothers' Views on Preparing Girls for Adolescence: A Qualitative Research.* 57th National Pediatrics Congress. 1. Rusy in Turkey Pediatrics Meeting, the 12th National Congress of Pediatric Nursing. 30 October-03 November 2013. Antalya (Poster First Prize).
5- Polat S, Bozok University, 2011 Scientific Publication Award (Third Prize in Health Sciences).

Publications from the Last 3 Years:
Alp Yılmaz F, Şener Taplak A, Polat S. Breastfeeding and Sexual Activity and Sexual Quality in Postpartum Women. *Breastfeed Med.* 2019 Jul 12. doi: 10.1089/bfm.2018.0249.
Gürol A, Tekgündüz K.Ş, Apay Ejder S, Polat S. Oral Glucose and Listening to Lullaby to Decrease Pain in Preterm Infants Supported with NCPAP: A Randomized Controlled Trial. *Pain Management*

Nursing 2019, 20; 54-61, DOI.org/10.1016/j.pmn.2018.04.008, (SSCI-SCI-Exp).

Kader O, Erbay A, Kilic Akca N, Alsac Yuzer S, Polat S. Hepatitis A immunization needs in nursing students in Turkey. *Tropical Doctor* 2018; 1-3, (SCI-Exp).

Alp Yılmaz F, Şener Taplak A, Polat S. Individual Applications of Turkish Lactating Women to Increase their Breastmilk Production. *Journal of Current Researches on Health Sector*, 2018; 8(2):121-134.

Akcan E, Polat S. The Effect of the Smells of Amniotic Fluid, Breast Milk and Lavender on Newborns 'Pain during Heel Lance. *Breastfeeding Medicine*. July/August 2016; 11 (6): 309-314, (SCI-Exp).

Kader O, Erbay A, Kilic Akca N, Polat MF, Polat S. Immunity of Nursing Students to Measles, Mumps, Rubella and Varicella in Yozgat Turkey. *AJIC American Journal of Infection Control.* (SCI-Exp), January 2016; 44 (1): Pages e5 – e7.

Polat S, Tufekci Guducu F, Kucukoglu S, Kobya Bulut H. Acceptance-rejection levels of the Turkish mothers towards their S children with cancer. *The Australian Journal of Nursing Practice*, Scholarship & Research (Collegian). April 2015; 23 (2): 217-223, DOI: 10. 1016 / j.colegn 2015.02.006, (SSCI-SCI Exp).

Polat S, Gurol A, Celebioglu A, Keskin Yildirim Z. The effect of therapeutic music on anxiety in children with acute lymphoblastic leukaemia. *Indian Journal of Traditional Knowledge*. January 2015; 14 (1): 42-46, (SCI-Exp).

Polat S, Ozyazicioglu N, H. Bicakci. Traditional practices used in infant care. *Indian Journal of Traditional Knowledge*. January 2015; 14 (1): 47-51, (SCI-Exp).

Ozyazicioglu N, Polat S. Traditional practices in Turkey: A literature review. *Indian Journal of Traditional Knowledge*. July 2014; 13 (3): 445-452, (SCI-Exp).

Gurol A, Polat S., Oran T. A qualitative study. *Journal Sexuality and Disability*. 2014; 32: 123-133, DOI: 10.1007/s11195-014-9338-8 (SSCI).

Polat S, Kucuk Alemdar D, Gurol A. Paediatric nurses 'experience with death: the effect of empathic tendency on their anxiety levels. *International Journal of Nursing Practice*. 2013; 19: 8–13, DOI: 10.1111 / ijn.12023, (SSCI-SCI Exp).

Aylaz R, Yilmaz U, Polat S. A qualitative study. *Journal Sexuality and Disability*. December 2012; 30 (4): 395–406, DOI: 10.1007 / s11195-011-9251-3, (SSCI).

Gurol A, Polat S. The effects of baby massage on attachment between mother and their infants. *Asian Nursing Research*. April 2012; 6 (1): 35-41, doi: 10.1016/j.2012/00.006, (SSCI).

Ayşe Şener Taplak, PhD

Affiliation: Assistant Professor, RN. Department of Pediatric Nursing, Yozgat Bozok University, Yozgat, Turkey

Research and Professional Experience: Child Health and Disease Nursing

Honors:
1- Şener Taplak A, Parlak Gürol A, Polat S, Polat M F. Forensic Cases Related to Children Reflected in the Media. International II. Forensic Nursing and I. Social Work Congress. 3-4 November 2016. Kırıkkale (Oral Presentation Award).
2- Polat S, Sener Taplak A, Daar G, Yuzer S. *Mothers'Views on Preparing Girls for Adolescence: A Qualitative Research*. 57th National Pediatrics Congress. 1. Rusy in Turkey Pediatrics Meeting, the 12th National Congress of Pediatric Nursing. 30 October-03 November 2013. Antalya (Poster First Prize).

Publications from the Last 3 Years:
Şener Taplak A, Erdem E. A Comparison of Breast Milk and Sucrose in Reducing Neonatal Pain during Eye Exam for Retinopathy of

Prematurity. *Breastfeed Med.* 2017 Jun;12:305-310. doi: 10.1089/bfm.2016.0122.

Taplak AŞ, Bayat M. Psychometric testing of the Turkish version of the premature infant pain profile revised-PIPP-R. *J Pediatr Nurs.* 2019 Jun 19. pii: S0882-5963(19)30035-1. doi: 10.1016/j.pedn.2019.06.007.

Alp Yılmaz F, Şener Taplak A, Polat S. Breastfeeding and Sexual Activity and Sexual Quality in Postpartum Women. *Breastfeed Med.* 2019 Jul 12. doi: 10.1089/bfm.2018.0249.

Alp Yılmaz F, Şener Taplak A, Polat S. Individual Applications of Turkish Lactating Women to Increase their Breastmilk Production. *Journal of Current Researches on Health Sector*, 2018; 8(2):121-134.

In: New Research on Breastfeeding ... ISBN: 978-1-53617-061-0
Editor: Kai Santos Melo © 2020 Nova Science Publishers, Inc.

Chapter 6

LONG-TERM IMPACTS OF BREASTFEEDING ON PREVENTION OF NON-COMMUNICABLE DISEASES

Motahar Heidari-Beni[1] and Roya Kelishadi[2],*

[1]Department of Nutrition, Child Growth and Development Research Center, Research Institute for Primordial Prevention of Non-Communicable Disease, Isfahan University of Medical Sciences, Isfahan, Iran
[2]Department of Pediatrics, Child Growth and Development Research Center, Research Institute for Primordial Prevention of Non-Communicable Disease, Isfahan University of Medical Sciences, Isfahan, Iran

ABSTRACT

Current evidence reported that non-communicable diseases (NCDs) including cardiovascular diseases, cancers, chronic respiratory diseases,

---

* Corresponding Author's E-mail: kelishadi@med.mui.ac.ir; roya.kelishadi@gmail.com.

and diabetes originate from early life. NCDs are usually caused by interaction of genetic factors, gender, age, ethnicity, environmental exposures, and lifestyle behaviors.

Breastfeeding is perfectly designed for the child's nutritional needs and it is the most advantageous feeding option for infants. In addition to its short-term benefits, it has several beneficial effects for prevention of NCDs for both mothers and children. Breast milk provides all the energy and nutrients that infants need for the first six months of life and is critical for sustaining the health of newborns and infants. Despite the beneficial effects of breastfeeding, it is still below the World Health Organization (WHO) recommendation in many countries.

Many studies showed long-term protective effects of adequate breastfeeding during infancy on NCDs particularly on hypertension, obesity, diabetes, dyslipidemia, and cardiovascular diseases at individual and population levels. However, there are controversial findings about these effects. Recall bias for exclusivity and duration of breastfeeding and low availability of infant nutrition data in retrospective cohorts may lead to inconsistent results between studies.

The primordial prevention of NCDs should start with an emphasis on improving breastfeeding practices. This chapter aims to summarize the current literature on the long-term effects of breastfeeding on prevention of NCDs and their risk factors.

Keywords: breast feeding, non-communicable diseases, risk factors

INTRODUCTION

There has been a dramatic increase in the prevalence of non-communicable diseases (NCDs) that is the cause of more than 60% of all global deaths and are forecasted to reach 69% by 2020 [1].

The most common of NCDs are heart disease, obesity, type II diabetes, cancer, immune diseases, chronic lung diseases, mental illness, chronic liver and renal diseases. Many of these diseases are linked to prenatal nutrition [2].

According to findings, genetics, gender, and age cannot be accountable for high prevalence of NCDs alone. Modifiable environmental and lifestyle factors also play an important role in the prevalence of NCDs [3]. Current evidence reports that occurrence of NCDs may be programmed by exposures during gestation or in the first years of life [4, 5].

Nutrition in early childhood including the type of milk can change disease susceptibility and therefore reduce the prevalence of NCDs. Focus on disease prevention in early life especially during first 1000 days (from conception through the first years of infancy) is logical and cost effective [6].

Breastfeeding is the first and most important source of nutrition for the infant that improves the survival, health, and development of all children [7].

Breastfeeding is less common in better-educated, wealthier, and urban women. Breast feeding substitutes were perceived as modern and prestigious. However, breastfeeding was correlated with being poor and unsophisticated [8].

Human milk contain bioactive factors including hormones, growth factors, neuropeptides, and anti-inflammatory and immunomodulatory agents [9]. It has long-term and short-term protection against diseases. It is well documented that breastfeeding has protective effects on infection diseases and lead to reduce the infant morbidity and mortality and increase infant survival rates [10].

Exclusive breastfeeding for six months after birth have been recommended by The World Health Organization (WHO). Breastfeeding can be continued for two years together with nutritionally-adequate complementary foods [11].

Levels of education, insufficient knowledge about benefits of breastfeeding, maternal race and ethnicity, breast diseases, insufficient production of breast milk, employment, duration of maternity leave, inadequate familial and health care professionals support are the main factors that prevalence and duration of breastfeeding [12].

Breastfeeding and Taste Preferences

Healthy taste preferences might be correlated with prevention of NCDs. Evidence has been shown that maternal diets during lactation affect taste preferences of infant. Different maternal diets lead to various ranges of flavors of breast milk. So, infants are exposed to a several range of taste which may influence later taste preferences [13]. Breastfed infants are more likely to consume foods and have healthier dietary patterns later in life. Children who receive breast milk, intake higher fruit and vegetables in later life [14].

Genetic, physiological, metabolic factors and specific taste molecules including T1R2, T1R3, and TRPM5 influence taste responses [15]. However, the association between the expression of these taste-sensing proteins and breast feeding has not been assessed. Effect of breast milk on taste preference may contribute to the long-term health benefits of breastfeeding [16].

Breastfeeding and Type I Diabetes

Breastfeeding lead to lower rates of obesity and diabetes compare with infant formula intake. Thus, the manifestation of the disease can be prevented by proper nutrition during the first months of life [17].

According to studies beneficial effects of breastfeeding are associated with duration of breastfeeding. A case-control study involving 1,390 preschoolers showed that receiving breastmilk for five months or longer play a protective role against diabetes (OR: 0.71, 95%CI: 0.54-0.93) [18].

Anti-infective properties of human milk lead to protective effect on diseases. Breastfeeding increases levels of T-cells and decreases levels of inflammatory cytokines including interferon, interleukin-4 and interleukin-10. However, these positive effects are inconsistent [19].

Meta-analysis on 17 case-control studies showed a weak effect between never having been breastfed (OR: 1.13, 95% CI: 1.04 to 1.23), infant formulas (OR: 1.38, 95% CI: 1.18 to 1.61) and use of cow's milk before 3 months of age (OR: 1.61, 95% CI: 1.31 to 1.98) and the risk of type I diabetes. These effects were observed in populations with low prevalence of breastfeeding not in populations with high rates of breastfeeding. So, differences in the prevalence of breastfeeding need to be investigated and considered in the design of case-control studies [20].

Assessment of 43 studies (two cohort and 41 case-control studies) showed that exclusive breastfeeding for more than two weeks reduced 15% the risk of type I diabetes [21].

Methodological problems related to the reliability of the data, the lack of details on breastfeeding duration, use of infant formulas and cow's milk, the age of introduction of complementary foods lead to different findings in studies [17].

According to findings, the type of feeding in the first year of life maybe associated with the development of chronic diseases with immunological etiology. Despite the inconsistency between results of the studies, increasing breastfeeding rather than cow's milk intake should be encouraged in the first year of life [17].

BREASTFEEDING AND TYPE II DIABETES

Breastfeeding is associated with lower risk of being overweight during childhood, adolescence, and adulthood. A meta-analysis on 39 studies published in the past 40 years that was conducted by WHO showed that breastfeeding correlated with less obesity in children (OR: 0.78, 95% CI: 0.72 to 0.84), even after adjusting for parental nutritional status, socioeconomic status, and birth weight. Therefore, breast milk protects against the development of obesity and consequently type II diabetes [22]. However, this association was not reported in some studies because of retrospective method to investigate the history of breastfeeding and the small sample size [23].

Biochemical constituents of breast milk and their differentiated nutritional composition lead to prevention of obesity and type II diabetes, promote the maturation of the immune system and reduce insulin resistance. Some bioactive substances affect energy balance and metabolic responses. Breast milk contains long-chain polyunsaturated fatty acids (LCPUFAs) including docosahexaenoicacid (DHA) and polyunsaturated fatty acids (PUFAs). These fats affect normal glycemic metabolism and number of insulin receptors in the brain of child [24]. Phospholipid skeletal muscle membranes of children that use breast milk have significantly higher amounts of DHA and other PUFAs than those without breast feeding. According to findings, low levels of DHA and PUFAs associated with insulin resistance. Formula-fed infants have high concentrations of basal and post-prandial insulin compared with breastfed infants that may lead to β-cell failure and type II diabetes [25]. However, there are inconsistence findings. Most of the studies were conducted in developed countries that mothers have high levels of education and income and pursue nutritional guidelines. Confounding factors can be identified by information from low and middle income countries because there is association between infant feeding practices and socioeconomic status [26].

BREASTFEEDING AND MORTALITY AND MORBIDITY

The ideal food for infants is breast milk that provides adequate energy and nutrients. Early breastfeeding initiation improves neonatal outcomes and must be universally recommended. Exclusively breastfeeding lead to only 12% of the risk of death compared with other feeding except breastfeeding [27]. Studies in low and middle-income countries reported that mortality increase 3.5 times in boys and 4.1 times in girls that were not breastfed [28].

According to meta-analysis of six high-quality studies, breastfeeding was correlated with a 36% (95% CI 19-49) reduction in sudden infant deaths [29].

According to findings of 3 prospective case cohort studies, there was 44% (95% CI: 20-61%) lower risk of all-cause mortality within 28 days among neonates that were fed by breast milk. Deaths from all causes among low birth weight neonates (42% lower [95% CI: 22-57%]) were also substantially lower among those exclusively breastfed within 24 hours [27].

According to WHO recommendation, exclusively breastfeeding for the first 6 months and continue until 2 years lead to save 800,000 children each year [28].

BREASTFEEDING AND OBESITY

It is difficult to accurately determine the prevalence and trend of obesity because of different criteria for obesity classification and the lack of age-adjusted data. However, there is no doubt that the prevalence of obesity in increasing in children and adults throughout the Asia-Pacific region [30]. Prevention especially during the childhood is so important. Breastfeeding and its longer duration have an important role in prevention of obesity and chronic disease. Breast milk, but not formula contains bioactive factors that have immunological, endocrine, development, neural and psychological benefits. It can control appetite in the neonatal period and infancy and influence in energy balance regulation in childhood and adulthood [31].

However, some studies did not confirm a critical role of breast milk. The results are often from observational studies, which can be changed by confounding factors including maternal age, level of education, maternal smoking, sedentary or physically activity lifestyle, maternal body mass index, race/ethnicity, parity, types of delivery, pregnancy complications, during pregnancy and infant health [32, 33].

So, because of controversial evidence and unclear underlying mechanisms, further researches are needed to increase knowledge and confirm the effect of breastfeeding on overweight/obesity [31].

113 studies reported that the odds of overweight or obesity reduced 26% (95% CI 22-30) with longer periods of breastfeeding [34].

Results of 23 high-quality studies with sample sizes of more than 1500 subjects reported breastfeeding lead to 13% (95% CI 6-19) reduction in the prevalence of overweight or obesity after adjustment for socioeconomic status, maternal BMI and perinatal morbidity [7].

Meta-analysis on 25 studies with a total of 226,508 participants from 12 countries showed that breastfeeding prevented obesity in childhood. The risk of childhood obesity was lower 22% in children that were fed by breast milk in comparison with those who were never breastfed [35].

The results showed that prolonged breastfeeding associated with reducing obesity risk. In particularly, Breastfeeding for more than 7 months can prevent obesity in later childhood. Further studies are needed to determine the effects of exclusive breastfeeding, exclusive formula feeding and mixed feeding on adiposity [7, 30].

The duration of breastfeeding is another factor that is important for decreasing the risk of obesity in later life. WHO and United States Department of Health and Human Services recommend breastfeeding for at least 6 months. Findings showed that duration of breastfeeding decreased the risk of obesity, hypercholesterolemia, hypertension and type II diabetes in later life. Short duration of breastfeeding associated with decreased appetite signaling and precocious introduction of solid food that contain more protein than human milk and finally correlated with obesity [31].

Longer duration of breastfeeding affects the fat mass and obesity associated (FTO) gene. The role of the FTO gene (SNP rs9939609 within the first intron) is increasing BMI and adiposity. Appetite regulation by hypothalamic, energy expenditure and metabolic rate can be altered by involvement of FTO gene. However, ability of breast milk to modify this gene has yet to be identified [36].

Assessment of 18 studies showed that breastfeeding greater than 40 weeks, was positively associated with a lower weight gain at 1 year [37].

Conversely, it has been showed that breastfeeding more than 8 months may have adverse effects including inhibition hypothalamic–pituitary–thyroid axis of newborn and increasing weight gain [38]. Moreover, other studies did not report significant relationship between risk of obesity and the duration of breastfeeding [38, 39].

Human milk contain several hormone molecules including insulin and insulin-like growth factor I (IGF-I), leptin, adiponectin, ghrelin, obestatin, and resistin. these hormonal molecules affect fat and lean body mass development in healthy term infants and increase satiety responsiveness of child and appetite signalling, and reduce the risk of over eating [31].

Another possible mechanism is the influence of breastfeeding on the establishment and modifies the development and maintenance of the gut microbiome. It has been shown that the composition of the gut microbiome is important in the development of some NCDs including diabetes and obesity. Lower counts of Bifidobacteria has been observed in faecal samples of obese children. Breastfeeding leads to increase the Bifidobacteria counts [30, 40].

Human milk has a moderate amount of calories and nutrients including carbohydrates, water, protein and fat and time and the diet of mother change its composition. However, formula contains higher levels of fat and protein than breast milk. Higher protein and fat consumption in early childhood have been correlated with obesity [35].

One of the main risk factor for many NCDs including diabetes, heart disease, and cancer is obesity. According to the World Cancer Research Foundation recommendation, all infants should be breastfed. Reducing the prevalence of obesity is one of the mechanisms of the effect of breast milk on cancer prevention [30].

BREASTFEEDING AND CARDIOVASCULAR DISEASES

Breastfeeding associated with decreasing cardiovascular risk factors. However, the effects of breastfeeding on cardiovascular diseases (CVD) are controversial. A systematic review did not reported any effect of breastfeeding on CVD mortality [10]. However, results of Nurses' Health Study showed that breastfeeding led to decrease the risk of CVD [41]. Recall bias for exclusivity and duration of breastfeeding and the lack of infant nutrition data in retrospective cohorts lead to inconsistent findings. More information related to the effect of breastfeeding on CVD is necessary [42].

BREASTFEEDING AND BLOOD PRESSURE

High blood pressure is positively correlated with the risk of stroke and ischemic heart disease. Studies have shown that NCDs progress and develop from early childhood and exposures in early life [43].

Breastmilk but not most brands of formula contain long-chain polyunsaturated fatty acids (LCPUFAs) including docosahexanoic acid (DHA) and arachidonic acid (AA). The major structural components of the vascular endothelium are LCPUFAs. Findings showed that LCPUFAs supplements decreased blood pressure of hypertensive adults [44].

DHA and AA synthesis is low in infants. So, the long-term effect of breastfeeding on blood pressure might due to its LCPUFAs levels. However, the long-term effect of LCPUFA supplementation on blood pressure in infancy is inconsistence. It has been reported that children who receive formula supplemented with LCPUFAs have lower blood pressure at 6 years compare with children who receive standard formula [45]. In contrast, another study reported that mean blood pressure levels were similar in children who receive formula supplemented with LCPUFAs and in a control group at 9 years. Socioeconomic and demographic factors as confounding led to different findings [46].

Obesity associate with hypertension. According to findings, breastfeeding prevent obesity so breast milk can protect against high blood pressure. Insulin-like growth factor 1 (IGF-1) is oppositely correlated with blood pressure in adulthood and positively related to breastfeeding. So, IGF-1 levels might be the potential mechanism of later blood pressure and breastfeeding [47].

BREASTFEEDING AND TOTAL CHOLESTEROL

Blood lipids levels are one of the main risk factors of Ischemic heart disease. Exposures in early life such as breastfeeding practices are associated with development of heart disease [48].

Long term blood cholesterol levels are affected by high cholesterol content of breast milk. Hepatic hydroxymethylglutaryl coenzyme A (HMG-CoA) is down-regulated by higher intakes of cholesterol in infancy and decrease the cholesterol synthesis. HMG-CoA reductase synthesizes cholesterol from acetate. HMG-CoA reductase inhibitors (statins) reduce the levels of cholesterol [49].

Findings showed that early exposure to high cholesterol levels was inversely correlated with later cholesterol levels. In addition, formula-fed animals had higher HMG-CoA reductase than milk fed animals [50].

CONCLUSION

Primordial and primary prevention of NCDs is important that mainly origin from early life.

The WHO and The United Nations Children's Fund (UNICEF) recommend exclusively breastfeeding should be initiated within 1 hour of birth and continue for the first 6 months of life. Infants should receive complementary foods with continued breastfeeding up to 2 years of age or beyond.

There are inconsistent results related to breastfeeding and prevention of NCDs. however, most studies have addressed the beneficial effects of human milk on health. Coordinated interdisciplinary strategies and further researches are needed to identify the exact mechanisms of breast milk on health.

REFERENCES

[1] Nyaaba GN, Stronks K, de-Graft Aikins A, Kengne AP, Agyemang C. Tracing Africa's progress towards implementing the Non-Communicable Diseases Global action plan 2013-2020: a synthesis of WHO country profile reports. *BMC Public Health.* 2017;17(1):297.

[2] Hanson M, Gluckman P. Developmental origins of noncommunicable disease: population and public health implications. *The American Journal of Clinical Nutrition.* 2011;94(6 Suppl):1754S-8S.

[3] Arena R, Guazzi M, Lianov L, Whitsel L, Berra K, Lavie CJ, et al. Healthy lifestyle interventions to combat noncommunicable disease-a novel nonhierarchical connectivity model for key stakeholders: a policy statement from the American Heart Association, European Society of Cardiology, European Association for Cardiovascular Prevention and Rehabilitation, and American College of Preventive Medicine. *European Heart Journal.* 2015;36(31):2097-109.

[4] Agosti M, Tandoi F, Morlacchi L, Bossi A. Nutritional and metabolic programming during the first thousand days of life. La Pediatria medica e chirurgica. *Medical and Surgical Pediatrics.* 2017;39(2):157.

[5] Koletzko B, Brands B, Grote V, Kirchberg FF, Prell C, Rzehak P, et al. Long-Term Health Impact of Early Nutrition: The Power of Programming. *Annals of Nutrition & Metabolism.* 2017;70(3):161-9.

[6] Schwarzenberg SJ, Georgieff MK. Advocacy for Improving Nutrition in the First 1000 Days to Support Childhood Development and Adult Health. *Pediatrics.* 2018;141(2).

[7] Victora CG, Bahl R, Barros AJ, Franca GV, Horton S, Krasevec J, et al. Breastfeeding in the 21st century: epidemiology, mechanisms, and lifelong effect. *Lancet* (London, England). 2016;387(10017):475-90.

[8] Rollins NC, Bhandari N, Hajeebhoy N, Horton S, Lutter CK, Martines JC, et al. Why invest, and what it will take to improve

breastfeeding practices? *Lancet* (London, England). 2016;387(10017):491-504.

[9] Andreas NJ, Kampmann B, Mehring Le-Doare K. Human breast milk: A review on its composition and bioactivity. *Early Human Development*. 2015;91(11):629-35.

[10] Geddes DT, Prescott SL. Developmental origins of health and disease: the role of human milk in preventing disease in the 21st century. *Journal of Human Lactation: Official Journal of International Lactation Consultant Association*. 2013;29(2):123-7.

[11] Kramer MS, Kakuma R. Optimal duration of exclusive breastfeeding. *The Cochrane Database of Systematic Reviews*. 2012(8):Cd003517.

[12] Balogun OO, Dagvadorj A, Anigo KM, Ota E, Sasaki S. Factors influencing breastfeeding exclusivity during the first 6 months of life in developing countries: a quantitative and qualitative systematic review. *Maternal & Child Nutrition*. 2015;11(4):433-51.

[13] Ventura AK. Does Breastfeeding Shape Food Preferences? Links to Obesity. *Annals of Nutrition & Metabolism*. 2017;70 Suppl 3:8-15.

[14] Anzman-Frasca S, Ventura AK, Ehrenberg S, Myers KP. Promoting healthy food preferences from the start: a narrative review of food preference learning from the prenatal period through early childhood. *Obesity Reviews: an Official Journal of the International Association for the Study of Obesity*. 2018;19(4):576-604.

[15] Beauchamp GK, Mennella JA. Flavor perception in human infants: development and functional significance. *Digestion*. 2011;83 Suppl 1:1-6.

[16] Beauchamp GK, Mennella JA. Early flavor learning and its impact on later feeding behavior. *Journal of Pediatric Gastroenterology and Nutrition*. 2009;48 Suppl 1:S25-30.

[17] Pereira PF, Alfenas Rde C, Araujo RM. Does breastfeeding influence the risk of developing diabetes mellitus in children? A review of current evidence. *Jornal de Pediatria*. 2014;90(1):7-15.

[18] Rosenbauer J, Herzig P, Giani G. Early infant feeding and risk of type 1 diabetes mellitus-a nationwide population-based case-control

study in pre-school children. *Diabetes/Metabolism Research and Reviews.* 2008;24(3):211-22.

[19] Piescik-Lech M, Chmielewska A, Shamir R, Szajewska H. Systematic Review: Early Infant Feeding and the Risk of Type 1 Diabetes. *Journal of Pediatric Gastroenterology and Nutrition.* 2017;64(3):454-9.

[20] Norris JM, Scott FW. A meta-analysis of infant diet and insulin-dependent diabetes mellitus: do biases play a role? *Epidemiology* (Cambridge, Mass). 1996;7(1):87-92.

[21] Patelarou E, Girvalaki C, Brokalaki H, Patelarou A, Androulaki Z, Vardavas C. Current evidence on the associations of breastfeeding, infant formula, and cow's milk introduction with type 1 diabetes mellitus: a systematic review. *Nutrition Reviews.* 2012;70(9):509-19.

[22] Owen CG, Martin RM, Whincup PH, Smith GD, Cook DG. Does breastfeeding influence risk of type 2 diabetes in later life? A quantitative analysis of published evidence. *The American Journal of Clinical Nutrition.* 2006;84(5):1043-54.

[23] Davis JN, Weigensberg MJ, Shaibi GQ, Crespo NC, Kelly LA, Lane CJ, et al. Influence of breastfeeding on obesity and type 2 diabetes risk factors in Latino youth with a family history of type 2 diabetes. *Diabetes Care.* 2007;30(4):784-9.

[24] Amatruda M, Ippolito G, Vizzuso S, Vizzari G, Banderali G, Verduci E. Epigenetic Effects of n-3 LCPUFAs: A Role in Pediatric Metabolic Syndrome. *International Journal of Molecular Sciences.* 2019;20(9).

[25] Abbott KA, Burrows TL, Thota RN, Alex A, Acharya S, Attia J, et al. Association between plasma phospholipid omega-3 polyunsaturated fatty acids and type 2 diabetes is sex dependent: The Hunter Community Study. *Clinical Nutrition* (Edinburgh, Scotland). 2019.

[26] Freitas HR, Isaac AR, Malcher-Lopes R, Diaz BL, Trevenzoli IH, De Melo Reis RA. Polyunsaturated fatty acids and endocannabinoids in health and disease. *Nutritional Neuroscience.* 2018;21(10):695-714.

[27] Debes AK, Kohli A, Walker N, Edmond K, Mullany LC. Time to initiation of breastfeeding and neonatal mortality and morbidity: a systematic review. *BMC Public Health*. 2013;13 Suppl 3:S19.

[28] Khan J, Vesel L, Bahl R, Martines JC. Timing of breastfeeding initiation and exclusivity of breastfeeding during the first month of life: effects on neonatal mortality and morbidity-a systematic review and meta-analysis. *Maternal and Child Health Journal*. 2015;19(3):468-79.

[29] Smith ER, Hurt L, Chowdhury R, Sinha B, Fawzi W, Edmond KM. Delayed breastfeeding initiation and infant survival: A systematic review and meta-analysis. *PloS One*. 2017;12(7):e0180722.

[30] Binns C, Lee M, Low WY. The Long-Term Public Health Benefits of Breastfeeding. *Asia-Pacific Journal of Public Health*. 2016;28(1):7-14.

[31] Marseglia L, Manti S, D'Angelo G, Cuppari C, Salpietro V, Filippelli M, et al. Obesity and breastfeeding: The strength of association. *Women and Birth: Journal of the Australian College of Midwives*. 2015;28(2):81-6.

[32] Anzman SL, Rollins BY, Birch LL. Parental influence on children's early eating environments and obesity risk: implications for prevention. *International Journal of Obesity* (2005). 2010;34(7):1116-24.

[33] Larque E, Labayen I, Flodmark CE, Lissau I, Czernin S, Moreno LA, et al. From conception to infancy - early risk factors for childhood obesity. *Nature Reviews Endocrinology*. 2019;15(8):456-78.

[34] Horta BL, Loret de Mola C, Victora CG. Long-term consequences of breastfeeding on cholesterol, obesity, systolic blood pressure and type 2 diabetes: a systematic review and meta-analysis. *Acta Paediatrica* (Oslo, Norway: 1992). 2015;104(467):30-7.

[35] Yan J, Liu L, Zhu Y, Huang G, Wang PP. The association between breastfeeding and childhood obesity: a meta-analysis. *BMC Public Health*. 2014;14:1267.

[36] Horta BL, Victora CG, Franca GVA, Hartwig FP, Ong KK, Rolfe EL, et al. Breastfeeding moderates FTO related adiposity: a birth

cohort study with 30 years of follow-up. *Scientific Reports.* 2018;8(1):2530.

[37] Buyken AE, Karaolis-Danckert N, Remer T, Bolzenius K, Landsberg B, Kroke A. Effects of breastfeeding on trajectories of body fat and BMI throughout childhood. *Obesity* (Silver Spring, Md). 2008;16(2):389-95.

[38] O'Tierney PF, Barker DJ, Osmond C, Kajantie E, Eriksson JG. Duration of breast-feeding and adiposity in adult life. *The Journal of Nutrition.* 2009;139(2):422s-5s.

[39] 3Neutzling MB, Hallal PR, Araujo CL, Horta BL, Vieira Mde F, Menezes AM, et al. Infant feeding and obesity at 11 years: prospective birth cohort study. *International Journal of Pediatric Obesity: IJPO: an Official Journal of the International Association for the Study of Obesity.* 2009;4(3):143-9.

[40] Simpson MR, Avershina E, Storro O, Johnsen R, Rudi K, Oien T. Breastfeeding-associated microbiota in human milk following supplementation with Lactobacillus rhamnosus GG, Lactobacillus acidophilus La-5, and Bifidobacterium animalis ssp. lactis Bb-12. *Journal of Dairy Science.* 2018;101(2):889-99.

[41] Rich-Edwards JW, Stampfer MJ, Manson JE, Rosner B, Hu FB, Michels KB, et al. Breastfeeding during infancy and the risk of cardiovascular disease in adulthood. *Epidemiology* (Cambridge, Mass). 2004;15(5):550-6.

[42] Wisnieski L, Kerver J, Holzman C, Todem D, Margerison-Zilko C. Breastfeeding and Risk of Metabolic Syndrome in Children and Adolescents: A Systematic Review. *Journal of Human Lactation: Official Journal of International Lactation Consultant Association.* 2018;34(3):515-25.

[43] Marmot M, Bell R. Social determinants and non-communicable diseases: time for integrated action. *BMJ* (Clinical research ed). 2019;364:l251.

[44] Stratakis N, Gielen M, Margetaki K, de Groot RHM, Apostolaki M, Chalkiadaki G, et al. Polyunsaturated fatty acid status at birth, childhood growth, and cardiometabolic risk: a pooled analysis of the

MEFAB and RHEA cohorts. *European Journal of Clinical Nutrition.* 2019;73(4):566-76.

[45] See VHL, Mori TA, Prescott SL, Beilin LJ, Burrows S, Huang RC. Cardiometabolic Risk Factors at 5 Years after Omega-3 Fatty Acid Supplementation in Infancy. *Pediatrics.* 2018;142(1).

[46] Pluymen LPM, Dalmeijer GW, Smit HA, Uiterwaal C, van der Ent CK, van Rossem L. Long-chain polyunsaturated fatty acids in infant formula and cardiovascular markers in childhood. *Maternal & Child Nutrition.* 2018;14(2):e12523.

[47] Khodabakhshi A, Ghayour-Mobarhan M, Rooki H, Vakili R, Hashemy SI, Mirhafez SR, et al. Comparative measurement of ghrelin, leptin, adiponectin, EGF and IGF-1 in breast milk of mothers with overweight/obese and normal-weight infants. *European Journal of Clinical Nutrition.* 2015;69(5):614-8.

[48] Oyri LKL, Bogsrud MP, Kristiansen AL, Myhre JB, Retterstol K, Brekke HK, et al. Infant cholesterol and glycated haemoglobin concentrations vary widely-Associations with breastfeeding, infant diet and maternal biomarkers. *Acta Paediatrica* (Oslo, Norway: 1992). 2019.

[49] Jiang SY, Li H, Tang JJ, Wang J, Luo J, Liu B, et al. Discovery of a potent HMG-CoA reductase degrader that eliminates statin-induced reductase accumulation and lowers cholesterol. *Nature Communications.* 2018;9(1):5138.

[50] Ronis MJ, Chen Y, Shankar K, Gomez-Acevedo H, Cleves MA, Badeaux J, et al. Formula feeding alters hepatic gene expression signature, iron and cholesterol homeostasis in the neonatal pig. *Physiological Genomics.* 2011;43(23):1281-93.

INDEX

A

adenosine, 77, 94
adiponectin, 52, 187, 195
adiposity, 72, 78, 91, 95, 128, 134, 186, 193, 194
adolescents, 75, 89, 92
amino acid, 30, 32, 48, 54
amniotic fluid, 154, 160, 161, 168
analgesic, 144, 150, 153, 155, 156, 157, 160, 161, 163, 164, 166, 167
antibiotic, 34, 46, 56
antibiotic resistance, 46
antibody, 29, 35
antidiuretic hormone, 149
antimicrobial therapy, 46
antioxidant, 32, 38, 39, 40, 41, 42, 53, 61, 66
antioxidative activity, 48
anxiety, 5, 13, 82, 86, 112, 119, 175, 176
apoptosis, 147, 164
appetite, 72, 74, 77, 90, 185, 186, 187
aspiration, xi, 142, 144, 145, 146, 149, 161
attachment, 11, 22, 111, 112, 176

B

bacteria, 34, 35, 53, 120
bacterial pathogens, 60
behavioral change, 112, 150
behaviors, ix, 70, 84, 87, 143, 146
beneficial effect, xii, 28, 29, 112, 180, 182, 189
benefits, viii, ix, xii, 6, 10, 15, 21, 27, 31, 55, 56, 70, 87, 107, 110, 112, 136, 144, 180, 181, 182, 185
bioavailability, x, 71, 72, 81, 82, 106, 115, 123
biochemistry, 48, 67, 68
biological activity, 28
biological processes, 48
biological responses, 11
biomarkers, 195
biotechnology, 68
birth weight, 83, 84, 85, 90, 91, 95, 117, 183, 185
births, 85, 112
birthweight, 91
blood flow, 76, 93

blood pressure, xi, 55, 134, 141, 147, 148, 188
blood urea nitrogen, 38
body mass index (BMI), 33, 37, 78, 86, 110, 185, 186, 194
bonding, 11, 12, 107, 112, 118, 119, 127, 128
brain growth, 6
breast cancer, 15, 23
breast feeding, 21, 92, 131, 133, 165, 173, 180, 182, 184
breast milk, v, vi, vii, viii, ix, xi, 9, 18, 25, 27, 28, 29, 30, 32, 33, 34, 35, 36, 37, 38, 39, 40, 41, 43, 45, 49, 51, 52, 53, 54, 57, 58, 61, 62, 63, 64, 71, 75, 76, 77, 79, 81, 82, 83, 87, 90, 91, 96, 97, 107, 115, 120, 127, 128, 137, 141, 142, 143, 144,150, 151, 152, 153, 154, 158, 159, 160, 161, 162, 164, 167, 168, 169, 170, 171, 172, 175, 176, 181, 182, 183, 184, 185, 186, 187, 188, 189, 191, 195
breast milk smell, xi, 142, 151, 153, 154, 161

C

caffeine, ix, x, 70, 74, 75, 76, 77, 78, 79, 87, 92, 93, 94, 95
calcium, 30, 35, 37, 42, 51, 106, 147
cannabinoids, 80, 81, 82, 84, 96, 97, 98
cannabis, ix, x, 70, 80, 81, 82, 83, 84, 85, 86, 87, 96, 97, 98, 100, 101, 102
carbohydrate(s), 29, 33, 55, 114, 147, 187
cardiovascular disease, xii, 179, 180, 187, 194
cardiovascular diseases (CVD), xii, 179, 180, 187
cardiovascular risk, 187
central nervous system, 6, 42, 74
cerebral blood flow, 147

child development, viii, 1, 2, 3, 4, 5, 7, 8, 9, 11, 17, 18, 23, 98
child mortality, x, 104, 120, 139
childhood, vii, ix, x, xi, 2, 5, 7, 19, 20, 70, 71, 77, 79, 88, 91, 95, 101, 113, 117, 120, 124, 134, 139, 141, 181, 183, 185, 186, 187, 188, 191, 193, 194, 195
Chinese women, 46, 64
cholesterol, 32, 125, 189, 193, 195
cigarette smoke, 72, 73, 99
cigarette smoking, 85
cognitive development, 3, 5, 6, 7, 8, 9, 12, 20, 21, 128
colostrum, 30, 33, 35, 41, 45, 49, 50, 52, 55, 56, 58, 61, 63, 107, 108, 109, 111, 112, 113, 163
consumption, 43, 51, 74, 77, 78, 81, 82, 84, 92, 93, 94, 147, 187
cytokines, 31, 55, 147, 182

D

demographic factors, 85, 188
developed countries, 15, 184
developing countries, 112, 123, 191
developmental milestones, 84
diabetes, xii, 15, 24, 35, 86, 101, 102, 180, 182, 183, 184, 186, 187, 191, 192
diarrhea, 112, 113, 119, 139
diet, 28, 30, 32, 36, 37, 38, 40, 56, 62, 94, 109, 113, 124, 143, 187, 192, 195
dietary intake, 107
digestibility, 108, 115
digestion, 31, 33, 34, 43, 54, 106
digestive enzymes, 29, 115
diseases, viii, xii, 4, 15, 18, 19, 34, 116, 117, 119, 179, 180, 181, 182, 194
dissociation, 48, 163
dyslipidemia, xii, 180

E

emotional, viii, 2, 4, 5, 8, 12, 13, 14, 15, 18, 37, 87, 107, 108, 112, 142
energy, xii, 13, 30, 32, 33, 36, 38, 55, 65, 74, 75, 92, 180, 184, 185, 186
enzymes, 31, 33, 35, 40, 52, 53, 54
epidemiology, 19, 89, 190
epigenetics, 3, 18, 25
epinephrine, 148
epithelial cells, 31
expressed breast milk, 151, 152, 158, 159, 160, 162, 170, 172

F

facial expression, 148
families, 3, 15, 112, 113
family history, 192
family members, 12
fat, 6, 30, 32, 33, 37, 40, 62, 72, 78, 81, 82, 94, 108, 116, 147, 151, 153, 162, 186, 187
fat soluble, 81
fatty acids, 6, 8, 32, 33, 56, 72, 107, 148, 184, 192
fetal development, 74, 85, 100
fetal growth, 74, 76, 78, 85, 102
fetus, 36, 76, 81
food, vii, x, 67, 68, 74, 81, 90, 92, 104, 105, 106, 107, 108, 109, 112, 118, 119, 123, 124, 137, 184, 186, 191
formula, 6, 8, 9, 12, 13, 17, 21, 29, 30, 31, 39, 40, 43, 44, 55, 56, 61, 66, 71, 72, 76, 115, 116, 119, 122, 127, 135, 136, 137, 154, 158, 182, 185, 186, 187, 188, 189, 192, 195

G

gastroenteritis, 112, 115, 120
gastrointestinal tract, viii, 27, 54, 65, 76
gene expression, 18, 77, 195
genes, 12, 19, 74
genetic diversity, 34, 53
genetic factors, viii, xii, 3, 180
genetic programming, 76
genetics, 25, 76, 181
gestational age, 31, 33, 54, 73, 86, 91, 101
gestational diabetes, 86
glucose, 33, 147, 148, 152, 155, 159, 164, 166, 167, 171
glutamate, 85, 147
glutamic acid, 54
glutathione, 40, 46, 48, 52, 53, 57, 64, 65, 128
glycans, 34, 53
glycoproteins, 34
growth, vii, ix, x, xi, 2, 4, 6, 8, 9, 28, 29, 30, 31, 32, 34, 35, 37, 38, 42, 51, 55, 57, 62, 64, 70, 71, 72, 76, 77, 78, 79, 82, 83, 84, 85, 86, 87, 88, 90, 91, 93, 94, 95, 100, 104, 106, 110, 115, 117, 120, 121, 124, 126, 134, 139, 142, 143, 146, 147, 148, 181, 187, 188, 194
growth factor, 29, 31, 35, 55, 72, 181, 187, 188
growth hormone, 72, 148
guidelines, xi, 75, 87, 107, 110, 142, 151, 184

H

health, v, vii, viii, ix, x, xii, 1, 2, 3, 4, 5, 10, 13, 15, 17, 18, 19, 20, 21, 23, 24, 27, 28, 34, 37, 51, 55, 58, 64, 66, 69, 72, 75, 77, 78, 80, 86, 88, 91, 99, 100, 102, 104, 105, 106, 107, 109, 110, 111, 112, 113, 117, 118, 119, 120, 121, 122, 123, 124,

125, 126, 127, 129, 130, 132, 133, 134, 135, 136, 137, 138, 139, 140, 161, 162, 172, 174, 175, 176, 177, 180, 181, 182, 185, 186, 188, 189, 190, 191, 192, 193
health care, vii, x, 104, 181
heart disease, 180, 187, 188, 189
heart rate, xi, 77, 141, 147, 148, 152, 153, 155, 160, 168
hemorrhage, 147, 149
hepatitis, 106, 167
herpes simplex, 106
heterogeneity, 105
high blood pressure, 188
hormone, 32, 74, 77, 82, 98, 187
hormone levels, 74
hormones, 29, 31, 52, 72, 115, 149, 181
human brain, 100
human development, 20, 58, 59
human health, 55, 122, 124
human milk, viii, 27, 29, 30, 31, 33, 34, 36, 37, 38, 40, 42, 44, 45, 46, 47, 49, 50, 51, 52, 53, 54, 55, 56, 57, 58, 59, 60, 61, 62, 64, 65, 98, 107, 108, 114, 115, 116, 120, 126, 128, 136, 162, 169, 182, 186, 189, 191, 194
human rights, vii, x, 104, 105, 107, 119, 126, 140
hypertension, xii, 149, 180, 186, 188
hypoglycemia, 33, 147
hypoxia, 74, 149

I

immune function, 98, 107
immune system, 4, 31, 35, 39, 51, 54, 123, 147, 184
immunization, 161, 165, 175
immunoglobulins, 29, 30
immunomodulatory, 181
immunomodulatory agent, 181
incubator, 117, 138

infancy, vii, ix, x, xii, 5, 54, 64, 70, 71, 72, 73, 74, 76, 77, 78, 79, 87, 88, 90, 91, 110, 113, 115, 143, 150, 180, 181, 185, 188, 189, 193, 194
infancy growth, 64
infancy weight gain, ix, 70, 72, 73, 90, 91
infant care, 113, 132, 175
infant feeding practices, 109, 135, 184
infant mortality, 4, 116, 117, 120, 139
infant nutrition, xii, 28, 45, 51, 57, 67, 105, 109, 121, 122, 124, 180, 188
infection, 2, 112, 149, 181
ingestion, 61, 76, 81, 82, 84, 93
insulin, 33, 55, 72, 147, 149, 184, 187, 192
insulin resistance, 33, 184
insulin sensitivity, 147
intensive care unit, 38, 43, 139, 162, 164, 168
intracranial pressure, xi, 141, 147, 149
intramuscular injection, 146, 151
intrauterine growth retardation, 96
iron, 35, 40, 42, 46, 48, 49, 60, 62, 106, 125, 195

J

jaundice, 46, 65

K

kidney(s), 76, 115
Kinsey, 102

L

lactation, 10, 15, 30, 31, 32, 33, 34, 35, 36, 37, 40, 41, 42, 43, 45, 47, 51, 54, 60, 61, 65, 77, 83, 84, 91, 99, 100, 109, 110, 112, 115, 119, 125, 128, 129, 132, 140, 182

Index

lactic acid, 35
Lactobacillus, 35, 194
lactoferrin, 30, 31, 35, 38, 40, 55, 57
lactose, 30, 33, 116, 150, 162
language development, vii, viii, 1, 6, 9, 10, 14, 18
leptin, 55, 72, 74, 77, 90, 94, 187, 195
lifestyle behaviors, viii, xii, 109, 180

M

macronutrients, 30, 32, 58
marijuana, 70, 96, 97, 99, 100, 101, 102
maternal smoking, ix, 6, 70, 74, 79, 90, 91, 185
meta-analysis, 6, 7, 17, 20, 23, 24, 61, 85, 90, 100, 125, 126, 183, 184, 192, 193
metabolic syndrome, 29, 55, 91, 94
metabolism, 33, 34, 59, 62, 76, 77, 93, 94, 184
metabolites, 56, 71, 72, 81, 82, 91
microbiota, 35, 54, 55, 56, 66, 106, 123, 194
micronutrients, 106, 123
milk quality, 134
molecular oxygen, 46
molecular weight, 48
molybdenum, 43, 48
morbidity, 4, 85, 101, 113, 129, 140, 181, 186, 193
mortality, 4, 112, 113, 117, 119, 129, 134, 137, 139, 140, 181, 184, 185, 188, 193
mortality rate, 4, 117
mortality risk, 4
motor behavior, 135
mRNA, 52
music therapy, 156, 171, 173

N

negative consequences, 107, 115

neonates, 43, 45, 46, 76, 128, 142, 157, 162, 164, 165, 167, 168, 169, 170, 171, 172, 173, 185
newborns, viii, xi, xii, 11, 27, 34, 39, 45, 47, 51, 59, 64, 65, 66, 83, 86, 90, 94, 107, 108, 109, 112, 130, 133, 141, 142, 144, 145, 146, 147, 148, 150, 151, 152, 153, 154, 155, 160, 161, 162, 163, 164, 166, 167, 168, 169, 170, 171, 172, 173, 175, 180, 187
nicotine, 71, 72, 87, 89, 90, 92, 107
nitrogen, 48, 54, 147, 148, 149
non-communicable diseases (NCDs), vi, viii, xii, 119, 179, 180, 181, 182, 187, 188, 189, 190, 194
non-enzymatic antioxidants, 39, 40
non-pharmacological methods, 143, 150, 168
nurses, 108, 109, 110, 113, 114, 116, 118, 119, 125, 126, 127, 176
nursing, 90, 106, 107, 109, 110, 111, 112, 113, 114, 117, 120, 125, 127, 130, 173, 174, 175
nutrients, xii, 2, 28, 29, 36, 37, 38, 46, 51, 57, 61, 64, 65, 106, 107, 115, 116, 122, 137, 144, 180, 184, 187
nutrition, vii, viii, ix, x, xii, 2, 27, 28, 29, 33, 36, 37, 38, 45, 51, 57, 59, 67, 87, 104, 105, 106, 109, 110, 112, 113, 117, 118, 119, 120, 121, 122, 123, 124, 135, 140, 180, 181, 182, 188
nutritional status, 107, 117, 183

O

obesity, ix, xii, 4, 18, 20, 35, 52, 70, 78, 79, 86, 88, 90, 95, 125, 180, 182, 183, 184, 185, 186, 187, 188, 192, 193, 194
obesity prevention, 88
omega-3, 192
opioids, 144, 151

overweight, ix, 70, 78, 86, 88, 90, 91, 95, 101, 183, 185, 186, 195
oxidation, 33, 41, 48
oxidative stress, 39, 46, 52, 148, 149, 171
oxygen, xi, 48, 141, 147, 149, 155, 157, 160, 169

P

pain, viii, xi, 141, 142, 143, 144, 146, 147, 148, 149, 150, 151, 152, 154, 155, 156, 157, 158, 159, 160, 161, 162, 163, 164, 165, 166, 167, 168, 169, 170, 171, 172, 173, 177
pain control, 150, 152, 163, 172, 173
pain management, vi, xi, 141, 142, 143, 150, 151, 161, 162, 164, 166, 168, 172, 174
painful procedures, xi, 141, 142, 143, 144, 146, 150, 151, 152, 153, 155, 158, 160, 163, 164
parenting, 3, 8, 9, 14, 16, 18, 21, 112
parenting behaviours, 3
parents, ix, 4, 5, 8, 9, 12, 16, 17, 70, 119, 140
pasteurization, x, 37, 40, 42, 43, 48, 56, 64, 104, 115, 116, 117, 119, 120
pathogens, 5, 34, 53, 106, 120
pathways, 2, 9, 72, 82, 142, 150
peer support, 17, 24, 25
pepsin, 54
peptides, 31, 32, 64
perinatal, 96, 101, 117, 119, 130, 132, 138, 186
polycyclic aromatic hydrocarbon, 83
polyunsaturated fat, 32, 58, 72, 184, 188, 192, 195
polyunsaturated fatty acids, 32, 72, 184, 188, 192, 195
postnatal exposure, 73, 74, 91, 100

pregnancy, ix, x, 8, 29, 49, 70, 71, 73, 74, 76, 78, 79, 83, 85, 86, 87, 88, 89, 90, 91, 93, 95, 96, 98, 99, 100, 101, 102, 109, 110, 112, 128, 131, 185
premature death, 114
premature infant, ix, 28, 29, 30, 36, 37, 40, 46, 51, 52, 54, 55, 56, 66, 118, 119, 138, 158, 160, 162, 171, 173, 177
premature infants, v, ix, 27, 28, 29, 30, 36, 37, 38, 40, 46, 52, 54, 55, 56, 59, 66, 118, 119, 158, 160, 162, 173
prematurity, 29, 31, 119, 158, 159, 163
preterm delivery, viii, 27
preterm infants, vii, viii, ix, 22, 28, 29, 30, 31, 33, 36, 37, 43, 46, 52, 57, 58, 59, 60, 61, 62, 63, 64, 93, 117, 119, 140, 143, 146, 147, 148, 149, 150, 153, 154, 158, 159, 160, 164, 166, 168, 171
prevention, viii, xi, xii, 35, 39, 88, 112, 113, 117, 139, 141, 180, 181, 182, 184, 185, 187, 189, 193
primordial prevention, xii, 179, 180
prolactin, 82, 98, 99, 107
proteins, 30, 32, 37, 48, 49, 52, 54, 61, 64, 144, 182
public health, 4, 5, 75, 88, 119, 120, 139, 190
pyridoxine, 128

Q

quality standards, 107, 115

R

race, 6, 86, 181, 185
radical formation, 46
radicals, 40, 60
risk factors, xii, 33, 86, 110, 180, 187, 189, 192, 193, 195

S

safety, 2, 37, 89, 92, 93, 107, 127, 167
saturation, xi, 141, 148, 155, 157, 160, 169
selenium, 42, 46, 48, 61, 63, 64, 65, 107, 128
sensitivity, viii, 1, 3, 7, 11, 12, 13, 18, 22, 23, 75, 147
serum, 30, 45, 47, 49, 52, 60, 63, 65, 97, 98, 99, 148
serum albumin, 30
skin, 3, 7, 11, 19, 22, 81, 112, 119, 133, 144, 156, 157, 161, 168, 169
skin to skin, 3, 7, 11, 19, 157, 169
smoke exposure, 90
smoking, x, 49, 70, 71, 72, 73, 74, 79, 87, 88, 89, 90, 91, 97, 99, 102, 110
smoking cessation, 88, 89
social inequalities, 113
social justice, 119, 120
social skills, 5
society, 8, 102, 113, 120
socioeconomic status, 46, 86, 183, 184, 186
sodium, 30, 42, 149
Solihull Approach, 16, 17, 23, 24, 25
stress, 5, 19, 37, 39, 52, 112, 119, 143, 147, 148, 149, 161, 170, 172
stress response, 148, 149
stressors, 17
stroke, 188
substitutes, 54, 115, 119, 120, 155, 181
sucrose, 152, 155, 156, 158, 159, 164, 166, 169, 170
sudden infant death syndrome, 4
supplementation, 33, 36, 37, 39, 46, 47, 51, 64, 128, 188, 194
survival, 2, 106, 114, 118, 121, 122, 133, 181, 193
survival rate, 114, 181
systolic blood pressure, 126, 193

T

therapeutic interventions, 146
therapy, 64, 89, 93, 156, 165
tobacco, 72, 74, 82, 83, 85, 86, 91, 99
tobacco smoke, 74, 82
toddlers, 125
toxic metals, 43, 49, 51
toxicity, 53, 81
toxicology, 80, 92
trace elements, 35, 42, 45, 48, 49, 51, 64, 65, 107

U

umbilical cord, 63
undernutrition, 115, 124
urine, 81, 90, 97, 98

V

venipuncture, 151, 154, 160, 161, 167, 169
ventilation, 149, 165
vitamin B1, 106
vitamin B12, 106
vitamin C, 46, 60, 62
vitamin D, 36, 37
vitamin K, 36
vitamins, 29, 35, 40, 107

W

water, 29, 39, 75, 105, 107, 112, 114, 115, 116, 149, 157, 158, 159, 187
water supplies, 112
weight gain, vii, ix, x, 56, 70, 71, 72, 73, 74, 76, 77, 78, 79, 84, 87, 88, 90, 91, 102, 119, 186, 187
weight loss, 132
welfare state, 139

World Health Organization WHO, viii, 1, 2, 4, 18, 19, 20 28, 30, 37, 66, 78, 107, 110, 112, 124, 126, 129, 130, 131, 132, 133, 134, 135, 136, 180, 181, 183, 185, 186, 189, 190

Z

zeitgeist, 13
zinc, 42, 47, 48, 51, 61, 62, 66, 106

Related Nova Publications

UTERINE FIBROIDS: EPIDEMIOLOGY, SYMPTOMS AND MANAGEMENT

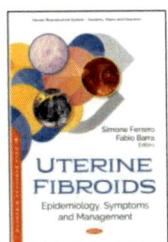

EDITORS: Simone Ferrero, MD, PhD and Fabio Barra, MD

SERIES: Women's Issues

BOOK DESCRIPTION: The aim of this book is to summarize the evidence regarding epidemiology, pathogenesis, clinical presentation, diagnosis and management of uterine myomas.

HARDCOVER ISBN: 978-1-53615-046-9
RETAIL PRICE: $195

WOMEN'S PEARLS

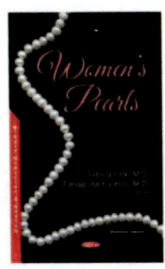

EDITORS: Sabina Fink, MD and Panagiota Korenis, MD

SERIES: Women's Issues

BOOK DESCRIPTION: *Women's Pearls* is a homage to women, as well as provides clinical pearls written by psychiatrists for clinicians and non-clinicians alike. Mental health as it relates to women is described throughout the chapters of this book. This book represents up-to-date information that can be used as a reference or as a study guide to understand clinical treatment for perinatal mental health.

HARDCOVER ISBN: 978-1-53616-103-8
RETAIL PRICE: $160

To see a complete list of Nova publications, please visit our website at www.novapublishers.com

Related Nova Publications

PERINATAL MENTAL HEALTH: CLINICAL MANAGEMENT HANDBOOK

EDITOR: Yoshiyuki Tachibana, MD, PhD

SERIES: Women's Issues

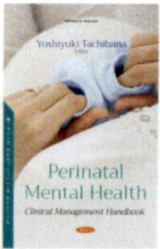

BOOK DESCRIPTION: Mental health problems often occur in perinatal periods. Mothers' mental health problems can cause parenting impairment and affect family health problems (e.g. child behaviors, cognitive development and physical health).

SOFTCOVER ISBN: 978-1-53615-774-1
RETAIL PRICE: $82

MATERNAL HEALTH: GLOBAL PERSPECTIVES, CHALLENGES AND ISSUES

EDITOR: Juan Sims

SERIES: Women's Issues

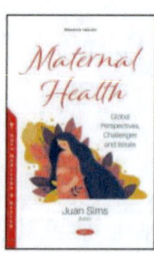

BOOK DESCRIPTION: In this compilation, a framework for exploring coupled physical-social systems impacts on health are presented. Specifically, this system is used to articulate three climate change impact pathways for maternal health: vectorborne diseases, water, sanitation, and hygiene, and nutrition.

SOFTCOVER ISBN: 978-1-53616-528-9
RETAIL PRICE: $82

To see a complete list of Nova publications, please visit our website at www.novapublishers.com